Localization of Brain Lesions and Developmental Functions

Fondazione Pierfranco e Luisa Mariani
viale Bianca Maria 28
20129 Milan, Italy

Telephone: +39 02 795458
Fax: + 39 02 76009582
e-mail: info@fondazione-mariani.org
www.fondazione-mariani.org

Localization of Brain Lesions and Developmental Functions

Edited by
Daria Riva and Arthur Benton

Mariani Foundation Paediatric Neurology Series: 9
Series Editor: Maria Majno

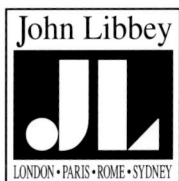

British Library Cataloguing in Publication Data

Localization of Brain Lesions and Developmental Functions
 – Mariani Foundation paediatric neurology series: vol. 9
 1. Brain – Diseases   2. Paediatric neurology   3. Child development
 I. Riva, Daria   II. Benton, Arthur L. (Arthur Lester), 1909   IV. Fondazione Pierfranco e Luisa Mariani

618.9'28

ISSN: 0969-0301
ISBN: 0 86196 599 X

Cover picture: Georgia O'Keefe *Red Hills, Lake George* 1927. The Phillips Collection, Washington DC

Published by

John Libbey & Company Ltd, PO Box 276, Eastleigh, SO50 5YS, England.
Telephone: +44 (0)23 8065 0208: Fax +44 (0)23 8065 0259

John Libbey and Company Pty Ltd, Level 10, 15–17 Young Street, Sydney, 2000, Australia.

© 2000 John Libbey & Company Ltd. All rights reserved.
Unauthorized duplication contravenes applicable laws.

Printed in Malaysia by Kum-Vivar Printing, 48000 Rawang, Selangor Darul Ehsan.

Contents

Chapter 1	Historical aspects of cerebral localization *Arthur Benton*	1
Chapter 2	The organization of memory in temporo-mesial structures in developmental age *Daria Riva, Veronica Saletti and Francesca Nichelli*	15
Chapter 3	Hemispheric specialization in acallosal children *Daria Riva*	23
Chapter 4	Interhemispheric communication in children with callosal agenesis *Daniela Brizzolara and Paola Brovedani*	35
Chapter 5	Acquired lesions of the corpus callosum *Giancarlo Tassinari*	41
Chapter 6	Basal ganglia lesions, language and neuropsychological dysfunction *Isabel Pavão Martins*	57
Chapter 7	Aphasic syndromes and localization of lesions in children *Philippe F. Paquier and Hugo R. van Dongen*	67
Chapter 8	The role of the left hemisphere in processing visuospatial information *Joan Stiles and Antigona Martinez*	79
Chapter 9	Contribution of frontal lobe lesions to cognitive deficit after closed head injury in children *Harvey S. Levin and Sandra B. Chapman*	97
Chapter 10	Agnosias *Francesca Nichelli and Daria Riva*	109

Chapter 11	Language in children with early brain damage: the development of brain-behaviour relations *Judy Snitzer Reilly*	121
Chapter 12	Non-verbal learning disabilities: development of the syndrome and the model *Byron P. Rourke*	133
Chapter 13	Congenital lesions of cerebellum *Francesco Guzzetta, Eugenio Mercuri, Maria Spanò and Maria Flavia Frisone*	145
Chapter 14	The cerebellum contributes to higher cognitive and social behaviour in childhood: evidence from acquired cerebellar lesions *Daria Riva*	151
	Index	161

Chapter 1

Historical aspects of cerebral localization

Arthur Benton

Department of Neurology, University of Iowa Hospitals and Clinics, Iowa City, IA 52242, USA

Dedicated to the memory of Justine Sergent

Summary

Thought and knowledge about the localization of mental functions in the human brain have a long and complicated history and are still evolving. There has been uncertainty about what the concept means, debate about where localization takes place and even denial that it exists. Ideas about cerebral localization have been determined primarily by the knowledge of brain anatomy existing at a particular time and by the availability of techniques for disclosing the presence and locus of brain lesions. They have also been influenced by concepts of the nature of disease and the prevailing state of psychological analysis.

This chapter presents a detailed analysis of the evolution of the concept of cerebral localization beginning with its earliest formulation (proposed about 300 AD) up to the present time, when the application of neuroimaging and cognate techniques to the question has forced a radical reevaluation of what 'localization' may mean. The pivotal developments of the nineteenth century, 'cerebral dominance' as a form of localization and the distinctive behavioural consequences of focal brain lesions in children are among the topics which are considered.

Experience is deceptive, judgement is difficult
Hippocrates, Aphorisms I, 1.

The evolution of the concept of cerebral localization of mental functions in the brain is a long and rather complicated story. There has been uncertainty about what the concept means; debate about where localization takes place and even denial that is exists. Ideas about cerebral localization through the ages have been influenced by the knowledge of brain anatomy existing at a particular time, by the availability of techniques for disclosing the presence and locus of brain lesions, by concepts of the nature of disease, by the state of psychological analysis, and perhaps even by the dominant technology of a period.

To begin, there was the question of whether or not the brain was in fact the organ of mind. Aristotle, the greatest of ancient philosophers and biologists, believed that it was not and he ascribed that important function to the heart. The heart was warm, the brain was cold and its primary function was to cool the animal and psychic spirits emanating from the heart. The heart moved, the brain did not. In excitement and emotional disturbance, the movements of the heart changed, the brain remained stationary. When the skull of an animal is opened, the brain is found to be cold to the touch and no movements are elicited when its surface is pressed. This cardiocentric theory of thought and emotion, reflected in so many familiar expressions in contemporary language usage, competed with cerebrocentric theory for over 2000 years, well into the 17th century (cf. Clarke, 1963; Gross, 1995).

The earliest form of cerebral localization, first proposed about 300 AD and accepted for 1500 years thereafter, placed the seat of mental processes in the ventricles of the brain rather than in its substance. The prevailing concept was that mental functions were carried by animal or psychic spirits through hollow tubes (called 'nerves') to the brain. Reaching the brain, these spirits gave rise to perception in the anterior ventricles. Proceeding to the third ventricle, the spirits produced reasoning or judgement. Proceeding further to the fourth ventricle, the products of perception and reasoning were stored in memory.

How did such an account, which today seems so bizarre, arise and why did it survive for so long a time? First, it was an expression of the dominant physiology and pathology of the period, which was humoral or fluid in nature. Health and disease were determined by the composition and condition of essential fluids that coursed throughout the body. Thus, ventricular localization can be seen as a specific application of the doctrine of humoral physiology that was accepted by physicians for more than a millennium through the Renaissance. Moreover, an empirical basis was claimed for ventricular localization. According to Bishop Nemesius of Emesia (ca. 350 AD), if the anterior ventricle is injured, sensation and perception are found to be impaired while intelligence and memory remain intact; if the third ventricle is injured, the mind is deranged; if the fourth ventricle is injured, there is loss of memory (cf. Telfer, 1955; Clarke & O'Malley, 1968). The tripartite division of mind into perception, intelligence and memory was a common formulation that was characteristic of medical thinking until 1800. Finally, we may note that ventricular localization was in accord with the dominant hydraulic technology of early European civilization, as reflected in the aqueducts and elaborate fountains that date back to ancient times.

But perhaps the main reason for the long life of ventricular localization is that, given the primitive state of cerebral anatomy before 1600, there seems to have been no viable alternative. While many mesencephalic and diencephalic structures – for example, the colliculi, the fornix, the thalamus and many others – were identified and named very early, the cerebral hemispheres were a *terra incognita*. No connections to or within them were known. As an early Renaissance anatomist looked at the surface of the brain, he saw a structure with innumerable loops and folds and lacking any systematic arrangement. It is not surprising then that the cerebral cortex was called the 'enteroid' or intestinal process (cf. Schiller, 1965). There seemed to be as little reason to name every pleat and fissure on the cortical surface as there would be to name every loop in the small intestine. It must be remembered in this respect that dissection of the human body was discouraged during the Renaissance. Consequently, the material at the disposal of anatomists was scant and of poor quality. As Renaissance anatomists examined the brain of an executed criminal it must often have been their lot to encounter decomposing cerebral hemispheres that had lost many details of their original form and that had the consistency and odour of spoiled cheese.

Chapter 1   Historical aspects of cerebral localization

Beginning in the 1600s, localization of mental functions in the substance of the brain gradually displaced ventricular localization. By this time autopsies were more frequently performed and microscopic study had indicated that the nerves were not hollow tubes through which the spirits could travel freely. Anatomists and clinicians placed the seats of perception, intellect and memory, in different structures – the corpus striatum, the corpus callosum, the white matter of the hemispheres and even in the cortex itself. For example, Thomas Willis, having placed perception in the corpus striatum and reasoning in the corpus callosum, regarded the cortex as a storehouse of memories. It is difficult to estimate the degree to which these localizations were speculative or, on the other hand, empirically grounded. However, in one instance at least, it is clear that clinical and experimental observations provided the basis for a specific localization. The 18th century French surgeon, La Peyronie, reported that in his clinical experience and from experimental manipulations, he found that only damage to the corpus callosum consistently produced mental derangement. Hence, reasoning '*à la fois par exclusion et grâce au fait*', he concluded that the corpus callosum was the seat of the mind (cf. Hécaen & Lanteri-Laura, 1977).

A radically different approach to functional localization was introduced at the beginning of the 19th century by that extraordinary figure, Franz Joseph Gall. As we know, Gall insisted that the cerebral hemispheres were not a homogeneous organ but an aggregate of about 30 specific regions, each of which was the 'organ' of a specific cognitive, emotional or social capacity. With the exception of his placement of organs for speech and verbal memory in the frontal lobes, his localizations, which ranged from the possible to the ridiculous, were generally not taken seriously by the scientific community. Nevertheless, his influence on subsequent thought was enormous for at least two reasons: first, he placed the seat of mental functions in the hemispheres; second, he proposed a scheme of mental functions that was far more differentiated than the traditional division into perception, reasoning and memory. There followed a spirited, at times rancorous, controversy between the 'localizationists' and the 'globalists' who on their part believed that the cerebral hemispheres acted as a unit.

However, more important than this controversy was the remarkable progress in cerebral anatomy that was achieved in the first half of the 19th century. Among other advances, the gyri and sulci of the superior, lateral and mesial aspects of the cerebral cortex were described and named, so that by 1860 illustrations of the cortical surface were essentially the same as those in textbooks today. During the same period and extending into the 1860s, the projection and association tracts were described in detail. These advances provided a firm anatomic basis for the intense interest and activity in functional localization that followed Broca's momentous discovery of the association between speech disorder and disease of the left frontal lobe.

The approach of clinicians and physiologists during the last decades of the 19th-century rested largely on the concept that the organization of the cerebral hemispheres consisted of a number of centres that harboured the memory images or representations of behavioural processes, together with their interconnections and their connections with lower levels of the brain. Clinical study and experimental manipulations led to the identification of these centres and their significance for behaviour and mentation.

Table 1 shows the localization of some of the cortical centres for speech and language that were postulated by leading investigators during this period. Each specific form of acquired language disability was ascribed to injury to a crucial aggregate of nuclei that was assumed to be the physical foundation of the intact ability. As Table 2 indicates, these precise localizations were not confined to language functions. Visual and tactile recognition, and spatial orientation, were also ascribed to the operation of focal cortical centres.

Table 1. Nineteenth century localizations: language centres in the left hemisphere

Centres	Locus	Result of lesion
Memory images of speech articulation (Broca, 1865)	Foot of third frontal gyrus	Broca's aphasia
Memory images of oral speech (Wernicke, 1874)	First temporal gyrus	Wernicke's aphasia
Memory images of writing movement (Exner, 1881)	Foot of second frontal gyrus	Agraphia
Visual memory of words and letters (Charcot, 1893)	Angular gyrus	Alexia
Memory for names (Mills, 1895)	Second temporal gyrus	Anomia

Table 2. Nineteenth century localizations: non-verbal centres

Centres	Locus	Result of lesion
Visual memory images (Wilbrand, 1897)	Parastriate region of occipital lobes	Visual object agnosia
Memory images of location (Dunn, 1895)	Occipitoparietal region of right hemisphere	Visuospatial disorientation
Memory images of tactile experiences (Wernicke, 1895)	Postcentral gyrus	Tactile agnosia

Yet during this 'golden era of localization' there were thoughtful students of the nervous system who objected to this placement of numerous cognitive capacities in sharply delimited cortical centres. They found it inconceivable that a restricted aggregate of nerve cells could be the seat of a complex intellectual function. Hughlings Jackson, who was well aware of the facts of clinical localization and applied them in his neurological practice, cautioned that identifying the lesion that leads to a neuropsychological disability was not the same as identifying the locus of the intact ability. In short, he accepted the concept of centres for its clinical utility, but not as a neuropsychological theory. Jackson's conception of the nature of aphasic disorder was also incompatible with the notion of cortical centres. He maintained that aphasia always entailed an impairment in intellectual functioning, a position that was diametrically opposed to that of Wernicke who insisted that there was no intrinsic connection between aphasia and intelligence.

One or another of Jackson's ideas was later expressed in the 1880s and 1890s by the physiologist, Jacques Loeb, by Sigmund Freud (then a neurologist as well as a psychiatrist) and by the philosopher, Henri Bergson. Their approach to the problem of localization in turn influenced the thinking of some early 20th century neurologists such as Arnold Pick, Henry Head and Kurt Goldstein.

But, on the whole, mainstream neurology remained wedded to the doctrine of cerebral centres and interconnected conduction pathways, the 'telephone system' conception of the functional organization of the brain. No doubt many neurologists regarded the concept of 'centres' as fiction. But it was a convenient and useful fiction. For example, Charion Bastian, a leading 19th century authority on aphasia, believed that the cerebral substrates of speech were, as he phrased it, 'diffuse but functionally unified nervous networks'. Nevertheless, he wrote that, while he did not accept 'the common conception of a neatly defined centre ... for the sake of brevity it is convenient to retain this word and refer to such networks as so many centres' (Bastian, 1898). The concept of centres was of heuristic value in clinical practice in that it pointed to the probable approximate locus of a suspected focal lesion.

Hemispheric cerebral dominance

Another quite different form of cerebral localization arose as a consequence of Broca's discovery, namely, hemispheric localization of mental functions. Today we accept without question that neural mechanisms in the left hemisphere are responsible for verbal and analytic cognitive processes. But in the 1860s the notion that a single hemisphere could be the seat of complex bilateral mental functions must have seemed so counter-intuitive as to be hardly credible. Broca himself called the idea 'subversive' and *'une révolution dans la physiologie des centres nerveux'* (Broca, 1863). It was only in 1865, after his own observations, as well as those of others, had established its truth beyond doubt that this brilliant yet cautious investigator proclaimed *'on parle avec l'hemisphère gauche'*.

At the same time a number of observations indicated that at least some left-handed patients with right hemiplegia were not aphasic and conversely that some left-handers with a left hemiplegia were aphasic. These findings, which linked hemispheric dominance for speech with hand preference, led to a symmetrical theory of hemispheric dominance which stipulated that right-handed persons were left-hemispheric dominant while left-handers were right-hemispheric dominant for speech.

All these observations were made on adult patients with documented or presumed unilateral hemispheric lesions. In 1868, only three years after Broca's pronouncement, Jules Cotard reported that children with congenital or early acquired atrophy of the left hemisphere were not aphasic. This was the first demonstration that cerebral organization in children was not necessarily the same as in adults.

Beginning in the 1870s and for several decades thereafter, the doctrine of left-hemisphere dominance continually expanded beyond the sphere of speech to encompass other cognitive functions. Jackson's ideas that the aphasic patient always suffered from some degree of intellectual impairment implied that the left hemisphere controlled at least certain aspects of thought. Finkelnburg (1871) characterized the defect as a loss of understanding of symbols, non-verbal as well as verbal, as in failure to grasp the meaning of graphic representations, insignia of rank and the like. The apraxia of Liepmann (1900) and the constructional apraxia of Kleist (1923) were ascribed to lesions in the left hemisphere. Marie (1906) insisted that 'true' aphasia represented a defect in intelligence and not merely an impairment in the ability to communicate. In brief, the left hemisphere became not only the speech hemisphere but also, as French neurologists were in the habit of calling it, 'the intellectual hemisphere'.

Throughout this period there were suggestions from time to time that the right hemisphere was also a significant mediator of mentation and behaviour. Both Hughlings Jackson (1878) and the German neuropsychiatrist Conrad Rieger (1909) advanced this idea, albeit in rather vague terms. Some ophthalmologists in the 1880s presented clinical evidence to support the idea that the right hemisphere played a special role in visuospatial performances, for example, in spatial localization of objects, route finding and geographic orientation. There was also Babinski's (1914) association of anosognosia with left hemiplegia and his speculation that a centre for the integration of somatosensory information with past experience might exist in the right hemisphere. However, in the face of seemingly overwhelming negative evidence, such as Dandy's (1933) report that complete extirpation of the right hemisphere had no appreciable effect on cognitive functions, these scattered findings were ignored and the right hemisphere remained the 'minor' or 'subordinate' hemisphere, devoid of any distinctive functional properties with respect to the mediation of behaviour. The most that could be said was that the right hemisphere might possess left hemisphere capacities in latent form, capacities that under some circumstances could be brought into play when the left hemisphere was damaged (for a review, see Benton, 1972).

The frontal lobes first became a prominent topic of clinical interest in the late 1880s when contributions by Jastrowitz (1888), Welt (1888) and Oppenheim (1890) described the personality changes, the peculiar behavioural features of trivial joking and gallows humour, and the disinhibition seen in patients with frontal lobe damage; Oppenheim called attention to the possible usefulness of this clinical picture as a sign of early frontal lobe disease. The experimental studies of Bianchi (1895, 1920–1922) on prefrontally ablated monkeys strongly supported these clinical findings of profound personality change and at the same time described these animals' loss of capacity to integrate experience in serial fashion. Decades later, in the 1930s, Jacobsen (Jacobsen, 1935; Fulton & Jacobsen, 1935) demonstrated personality changes in the direction of passivity and equanimity in prefrontally ablated chimpanzees and, in addition, by means of the delayed response task, described a specific deficit in the capacity to retain representations over time. A brief contribution by the French surgeon Clovis Vincent (1936) emphasized the importance of the connections to the frontal lobes in producing behaviour change; at the same time, he discounted the effects of damage within the prefrontal region itself, arguing for a connectionist or network concept of frontal lobe functioning.

The period between the two world wars (1920–1940) saw divergent trends with respect to localization. On the one hand, extremely detailed cortical maps, calling for the placement of 40 to 80 functions, were developed by Henschen (1922), Kleist (1934) and Nielsen (1936). They were not widely accepted. On the other hand, there was a definite waning of interest in problems of localization in favour of analyses of the basic nature of the language and perceptual disorders exhibited by patients with brain disease. Head (1926), the most prominent aphasiologist of the time, argued that aphasia was an expression of a general impairment in symbolic thinking that manifested itself in defective non-verbal as well as verbal performances. Kurt Goldstein (1934) proposed a holistic theory of brain function according to which even a focal lesion produces a general alteration of mentation and behaviour. He laid great stress on what he termed loss of the 'abstract attitude', which can be viewed as a forerunner of the concept of 'executive functions' in contemporary neuropsychology.

During these interwar years there was a burgeoning of interest in the effects of early brain damage, a development that was stimulated by a number of factors, among them the pandemic of encephalitis lethargica in the 1920s which left thousands of non-defective brain-damaged children in its wake, and also advances in paediatric care which resulted in the survival of low birthweight developmentally disabled infants. The hyperactivity and aggressiveness which were characteristic of many post-encephalitic children were often ascribed to disinhibition produced by frontal lobe dysfunction.

Orton (1925) advanced the concept that developmental dyslexia, as well as other disorders such as stuttering and motor awkwardness, were expressions of an incomplete establishment of hemispheric specialization of function. The implications of his highly original contribution are still being explored today. Equally important were the ablation studies of Kennard (1938, 1940) on infant monkeys that purported to show that experimentally produced focal lesions did not lead to the motor deficits that followed similar lesions in adult animals. This early exploration forcefully raised the question of the plastic character of the immature brain and marked the beginning of this major area of research on both animals and human subjects which has been so intensively investigated in recent decades.

In the decades following World War II there was an extraordinary increase of interest in brain function and brain-behaviour relationships. Advances in neuroanatomy and neuropharmacology, the development of more incisive methods of neuropsychological assessment, which largely displaced the impressionistic evaluations of earlier times, and increased sophistication in the design of studies provided a sound basis for this expansion. Without doubt the unprecedented governmental support of scientific research in the area, first in the United States and later in Europe as it recovered from the ravages of the war, was also a decisive factor.

The advances that were achieved in the 1950s and 1960s were many and varied. Only a few that clearly opened new possibilities and changed the direction of thinking can be mentioned: the demonstration by Scoville & Milner (1957) of the crucial role of the hippocampus in learning and memory; the study of hemispheric specialization for speech in left-handers by Goodglass & Quadfasel (1954) which showed that the simple 'mirror-image' concept was incorrect and that the real situation was rather more complex. Geschwind's (1965) analysis of the aphasic, agnostic and apraxic disorders, his demonstration of the morphological differences between the left and right hemispheres (Geschwind & Levitsky, 1968) and his neo-connectionist theory of brain function forcefully returned anatomy to the study of higher-level mental impairments and inspired a large body of research along these lines. Still another significant advance was the quantitative assessment of fluent and aphasic speech and its correlation with locus of lesion that was developed by the Boston aphasia school (cf. Goodglass *et al.*, 1964, Benson, 1967).

The most important change in our conception of the differences between the two cerebral hemispheres was initiated by the studies of Hécaen (Hécaen *et al.*, 1951, 1956) and Zangwill (McFie *et al.*, 1950) and their co-workers which demonstrated conclusively that patients with right-hemisphere disease show a very high frequency of specific visuoperceptual, visuospatial and visuoconstructional defects. Thus, the scattered findings of earlier investigators were confirmed. In effect these studies, indicating that the right hemisphere also possessed distinctive functional properties in the mediation of behaviour, invalidated the doctrine of exclusive left-hemisphere dominance and put in its place the more egalitarian concept of asymmetry of hemispheric function.

The Hécaen-Zangwill initiative had a number of consequences. Its implications led to a widespread exploration of the role that the right hemisphere might be playing in the mediation of various aspects of mentation. The result was that a remarkably diverse array of capacities and attributes, far beyond the visuoperceptual and visuoconstructional abilities described by Hécaen and Zangwill, were ascribed to operations in the right hemisphere. A list of these is shown in Table 3. As will be seen, in addition to sensory and motor functions, the inventory includes attentional processes, level of awareness, and affective reactivity. It was obvious that a simple verbal vs. non-verbal dichotomy could not account for these presumed differences in hemispheric specialization, and a number of other cognitive dimensions were proposed, as shown in Table 4. But taken singly, none of these was more adequate than the verbal–non-verbal dichotomy and finally the suggestion was made that a multi-dimensional criterion might be the answer.

Table 3. Performances mediated by right hemisphere

Vision
Discrimination of configurations (e.g. complex shapes)
Spatial orientation (e.g. route finding, directions, geography)
Recognition of familiar faces, unfamiliar faces, facial expression
Stereopsis
Mental rotation

Audition
Sound localization
Discrimination of pitch, loudness, timbre
Perception of emotional oral speech
Identification of persons by voice
Understanding of metaphoric speech

Somesthesis
Object and form perception
Perception of spatial stimuli (e.g. direction of lines drawn on skin)

Motor
Simple reaction time
Music: instrumental performance
Singing
Prosody in speech
Motor persistence

General
Arousal and attention
Preparatory set
Awareness of hemispace
Mood (euphoria/dysphoria)

Table 4. Left hemisphere/right hemisphere dichotomies

Verbal vs. non-verbal	Logical vs. pictorial
Serial vs. parallel	Propositional vs. appositional
Analytic vs. holistic	Rational vs. intuitive
Controlled vs. creative	Social vs. physical

However, it also became evident that the specialization of the right hemisphere for any function was not nearly as sharp as was the specialization of the left hemisphere for language. The studies of Conrad (1949) and Russell & Espir (1961) on right-handed soldiers who had been rendered aphasic by penetrating wounds apparently confined to a single hemisphere confirmed what had long been assumed, namely, that 'crossed' aphasia (i.e. produced by a right hemisphere lesion in a right-handed patient) was a rare occurrence. In Conrad's study the observed frequency was 6 per cent and in the better controlled study of Russell & Espir it was 1.8 per cent. But when the same analysis was applied to disabilities associated with lesions of the right hemisphere, the findings were rather different. Studies by Arrigoni & De Renzi (1964) and Benton (1967) found that the frequency of 'crossed' constructional apraxia in right-handed patients with *left* hemisphere lesions was 32 per cent and 28 per cent, respectively. Similarly, Benton & Van Allen (1968), investigating impairment in facial recognition in patients with unilateral disease, found that 23 per cent had *left* hemisphere lesions.

These observations showed that, although there was indeed asymmetry of hemispheric function, this asymmetry was itself asymmetric, so to speak, with a much more clear specialization of function in the left hemisphere than in the right. Later studies of normal subjects added other dimensions to the topic. Employment of the dichotic listening procedure and of tachistoscopic visual half-field stimulation disclosed considerable instability in their performances from one testing session to another and even within the course of a single testing session (cf. Pizzamiglio *et al.*, 1974; Blumstein *et al.*, 1975; Turkewitz & Ross, 1983). Specific instructions and duration of stimulus exposure were also found to be significant determinants of the degree of differential hemispheric participation in a performance like facial recognition (cf. Galper & Costa, 1980). These indications of flexibility in function and inter-hemispheric communication in normal subjects could not help but raise doubts about the validity of simple interpretations of the defective performances of patients with unilateral brain disease.

The 1950s were the heyday of the surgical operation of prefrontal leukotomy when tens of thousands of psychiatric patients were subjected to that 'great and desperate cure' (Valenstein, 1986). The therapeutic effects of the intervention were minimal but it did yield some useful information about frontal lobe functioning. Autopsy study of patients who had died after surgery clarified the arrangement of prefrontal-thalamic connections in the human brain. Behavioural findings largely confirmed earlier observations but also disclosed many instances in which no appreciable changes in cognition or personality could be detected (for reviews, see Benton, 1991, 1994).

Investigation of organically-based cognitive disabilities and behaviour disorders in children showed a remarkable growth during these early post-war decades. Reading disability (renamed developmental dyslexia to emphasize organic determinants as compared to educational or psychogenic causation) was investigated intensively through electroencephalography, evaluation of 'soft' neurological signs and the identification of specific perceptual defects that were presumed to be indicative of cerebral maldevelopment (for a review, see Benton, 1975). The diagnostic category of 'minimal brain damage' arose to cover a myriad of diverse behavioural abnormalities including hyperactivity, aggression (and its opposite, passivity), impulsivity, disturbances of attention, motor awkwardness and learning disabilities. Criticized as being neurologically meaningless. the concept nevertheless reflected the conviction of clinicians that what was wrong with these children could not be attributed to faulty nurture or psychological conflict.

There was little direct study of localization of cerebral function in children for the simple reason that suitable case material was not available. Ischaemic infarcts, the optimal type of lesion for assessing the psychological effects of focal brain lesions, are rare in children and the more frequent types of injury (i.e. trauma and infection) were not useful for the purpose in that pre-neuroimaging era. However, there was much interest in the development of hemispheric specialization and in the plasticity of the immature brain, both of which topics had clear implications for localization of function.

For example, the recovery of speech after brain damage was a fertile field of investigation. The aphasia exhibited by children who had sustained brain injury showed some distinctive characteristics, in that it was of the nonfluent expressive type with an impoverished lexicon, with somewhat better understanding of oral speech and lacking the semantic paraphasias and logorrhea of adult patients with Wernicke aphasia. Muteness, an uncommon finding in adult aphasics, was very frequent. The assertion was made that impairment of verbal functions was likely to occur independently of which hemisphere bore the brunt of the damage (cf. Basser, 1962). Above all, emphasis was placed on the more rapid and more complete recovery from aphasic disorder in children as compared to adults. A negative linear relationship between age at injury and degree of recovery was also postulated. However, these generalizations were significantly modified in the light of later investigative work that examined the issues more critically and disclosed less optimistic outcomes of childhood brain injury (for reviews, see St. James Roberts, 1979; Levin *et al.*, 1984; Spreen *et al.*, 1995).

Retrospect

We may take a look at the interpretations and conclusions of our predecessors and make an assessment in the light of our present understanding. Some have stood the test of time reasonably well, at least in a broad sense, while some have not. With respect to the aphasic disorders, for example, the precise placement of centres for nonfluent and fluent speech has had to be modified. Broca's aphasia is produced by a more extensive lesion in the posterior frontal and anterior temporal territory than was previously thought (cf. Vignolo, 1988; Damasio, 1989, 1991; Damasio, 1992; Benson, 1993). A lesion which is strictly limited to Broca's area most often leads only to a transient impairment in expressive speech, and sometimes none at all. As it happens, a judicious reading of early neurosurgical observations might have led to the same conclusion. The pioneer psychosurgeon, Burckhart (1891) reported that partial excision of Broca's area in hospitalized psychotic patients led only to a transient expressive speech disturbance and the same result was found by Dandy (1922) in his operated tumour cases.

Studies of patients with Wernicke's aphasia have produced similar, but not quite identical findings. There is no doubt that a lesion confined to Wernicke's area can lead to the disorder. More often the causative lesion proves to be one involving Wernicke's area and surrounding territory. Moreover an occasional case of a 'silent' lesion in Wernicke's area as well as of chronic Wernicke patients with lesions sparing Wernicke's area also have been described (cf. Boller, 1973; Dronkers *et al.*, 1995).

A word of caution at this point is perhaps appropriate. We evaluate earlier ideas from a vantage point that has benefited from the carefully designed investigative work of recent decades, from more refined techniques of mental measurement and, above all, from those remarkable neuroimaging procedures, such as CT and MRI, that have given us the opportunity to enhance our understanding of brain-behaviour relationships to a degree that was scarcely imaginable 30 years ago. However, as authorities in this area have emphasized, the generation of valid neuroimaging data and their correct interpretation are extremely complex tasks (cf. Vignolo, 1988; H. Damasio, 1995; Nadeau & Crosson, 1995). Hanna Damasio in particular has detailed the numerous pitfalls that inevitably lead to incorrect conclusions about lesional localization. The point that must be made is that these pitfalls are not yet generally recognized by clinicians and researchers with the result that many reports in the current literature cannot be accepted at face value. No doubt this state of affairs will improve in future years but as of today published neuroimaging findings are not quite the 'gold standard' that many of us have assumed them to be.

As one surveys the evolution of localization theory through the ages, one cannot help but note that, as in so many fields of science and scholarship, there has been a progression from the simple to the complex. Specifically, there has been an evolution of concepts of cerebral organization from hydraulic systems to reflex arcs to telephone circuits to today's neural network models. There has been a progression in behavioural analysis from the tripartite classification of perception, reasoning and memory through faculty and multiple abilities psychology to the component processes postulated in contemporary cognitive psychology. In the field of aphasia there has been the evolution from the unitary 'speechlessness' of Hippocratic medicine through the distinction between fluent and nonfluent types of speech disorder to the diagnostic categories of the late 19th century clinicians; now modern aphasiological study shows that these categories (e.g. Broca's aphasia and Wernicke's aphasia) need to be fractionated if progress in the localization of language functions is to be achieved. There is the evolution of the concept of left-handedness as the opposite of right-handedness to the present uncertainty about what its neuropsychological implications are. Finally, there has been a progression from the assumption of a clear differentiation of functions between the hemispheres to the more complicated concept of interhemispheric interaction and integration.

This historical process of transmutation from the simple to the complex necessarily has brought with it an increased difficulty in the analysis and interpretation of observations relevant to the question of cerebral localization. The Hippocratic aphorism at the head of this chapter characterizes the present state of affairs, in which investigators attempt to interpret complex computer-generated mathematically transformed data, as aptly as it reflected the situation 2400 years ago. Judgement *is* difficult and clinical and experimental findings *are* often misleading. Neuroscientists concerned with functional localization in the human brain face a very formidable challenge. When the questions inherent in that challenge are answered satisfactorily we will have a deeper understanding of what 'localization' really means and be able to utilize that understanding in the clinic.

References

Arrigoni, G. & De Renzi, E. (1964): Constructional apraxia and hemispheric locus of lesion. *Cortex* **1,** 170–197.

Babinski, J. (1914): Contribution à l'étude des troubles mentaux dans l'hémiplégie organique cérébrale (anosagnosie). *Rev. Neurol.* **22,** 845–848.

Basser, L.S. (1962): Hemiplegia of early onset and the faculty of speech with special reference to the effects of hemispherectomy. *Brain* **85,** 427–460.

Bastian, H.C. (1898): *A treatise on aphasia and other speech defects*. New York: Appleton.

Benson, D.F. (1967): Fluency in aphasia: correlation with radioactive scan localization. *Cortex* **3,** 373–394.

Benson, D.F. (1993): Aphasia. In: *Clinical neuropsychology*, 3rd edn., eds. K.M. Heilman & E. Valenstein. New York: Oxford University Press.

Benton, A.L. (1967): Constructional apraxia and the minor hemisphere. *Confinia Neurologica* **29**, 1–16.

Benton, A.L. (1972): The 'minor' hemisphere. *J. Hist. Med. Allied Sci.* **27**, 5–11.

Benton, A.L. (1975): Developmental dyslexia: neurological aspects. *Adv. Neurol.* **7**, 1–47.

Benton, A.L. (1991): The prefrontal region: its early history. In: *Frontal lobe function and dysfunction*, eds. H.S. Levin, H.M. Eisenberg & A.L. Benton. New York: Oxford University Press.

Benton, A.L. (1994): The frontal lobes: a historical sketch. In: *Handbook of neuropsychology*, eds. F. Boller, H. Spinnler & J.A. Hendier, **9**, pp. 3–16. Amsterdam: Elsevier.

Bianchi, L. (1895): The functions of the frontal lobes. *Brain* **18**, 497–522.

Bianchi, L. (1920): *La meccanica del cervello e la funzione dei lobi frontali*. Turin: Brocca. English translation by J.H. Macdonald. *The mechanism of the brain*. Edinburgh: Livingston, 1922.

Blumstein, S., Goodglass, H. & Tartter, V. (1975): The reliability of ear advantage. *Brain Lang.* **2**, 226–236.

Boller, F. (1973): Destruction of Wernicke's area without language disturbance. *Neuropsychologia* **11**, 243–246.

Broca, P. (1863): Localisation des fonctions cérébrales: siège du langage articulé. *Bull. Soc. d'Anthropologie* **6**, 200–204.

Burckhardt, G. (1891): Ueber Rindenexcisionen als Beitrag der operativen Therapie der Psychosen. *Allgemeine Zeitschrift für Psychiatrie* **47**, 463–548.

Clarke, E. (1963): Aristotelian concepts of the form and function of the brain. *Bull. Hist. Med.* **37**, 1–14.

Clarke, E. & O'Malley, C.D. (1968): *The human brain and spinal cord*. Berkeley: University of California Press.

Conrad, K. (1949): Ueber aphasischer Sprachstoerungen bei Linkshaendern. *Nervenarzt* **20**, 148–154.

Damasio, A.R. (1992): Aphasia. *New Eng. J. Med.* **326**, 531–539.

Damasio, H. (1989): Neuroimaging contributions to the understanding of aphasia. In: *Handbook of neuropsychology*, eds. F. Boller & J. Grafman, **2**. Amsterdam: Elsevier.

Damasio, H. (1991): Neuroanatomical correlates of the aphasias. In: *Acquired aphasia*, 2nd edn., ed. M.T. Sarno. New York: Academic Press.

Damasio, H. (1995): *Human brain anatomy in computerized images*. New York: Oxford University Press.

Dandy, W.E. (1922): Treatment of non-encapsulated brain tumors by extensive resection of contiguous brain tissue. *Bull. Johns Hopkins Hospital* **33**, 188.

Dandy, W.E. (1933): Physiological studies following extirpation of the right cerebral hemisphere in man. *Bull. Johns Hopkins Hospital* **53**, 31–51.

Dronkers, N.F., Redfern, B.B. & Ludy, C.A. (1995): Lesion localization in chronic Wernicke's aphasia. *Brain Lang.* **51**, 62–65.

Finkelnberg, F.C. (1871): Niederrheinische Gesellschaft: Sitzung von 21 Maerz 1870 in Bonn. *Berliner Klinische Wochenschrift* **7**, 449–450.

Fulton, J.F. & Jacobsen, C.F. (1935): The functions of the frontal lobes. *Abstracts, Second International Neurological Congress* **2**, 70–71. London.

Galper, E. & Costa, L. (1980): Hemispheric superiority for recognizing faces depends upon how they are learned. *Cortex* **16**, 21–38.

Geschwind, N. (1965): Disconnection syndromes in animals and man. *Brain* **88**, 237–294; 585–644.

Geschwind, N. & Levitsky, W. (1968): Human brain: left-right asymmetries in temporal speech region. *Science* **161**, 186–187.

Goldstein, K. (1934): *Der Aufbau des Organismus*. Den Haag: Nijhoff. English translation: *The Organism*. New York: American Book Company (1939).

Goodglass, H. & Quadfasel, F. (1954): Language laterality in left-handed aphasics. *Brain* **77**, 521–548.

Goodglass, H., Quadfasel, F. & Timberlake, W.H. (1964): Phrase length and type and severity of aphasia. *Cortex* **1**, 133–153.

Gross, C.G. (1995): Aristotle on the brain. *The Neuroscientist* **1**, 245–250.

Head, H. (1926): *Aphasia and kindred disorders of speech*. London: Cambridge University Press.

Hécaen, H., Ajuriaguerra, J. & Massonet, J. (1951): Les troubles visuoconstructifs par lésion pariéto-occipitale droite. *Encéphale* **40**, 122–179.

Hécaen, H. & Lanteri-Laura, G. (1977): *Evolution des connaissances et des doctrines sur les localisations cérébrales*. Paris: Desclée de Brouwer.

Hécaen, H., Penfield, W., Bertand, C. & Malmo. R. (1956): The syndrome of apractagnosia due to lesions of the minor hemisphere. *Arch. Neurol. Psychiat.* **75**, 400–434.

Henschen, S.E. (1992): *Klinische und Anatomische Beitraege zur Pathologie des Gehirns*. Stockholm: Nordisk Bokhandeln.

Jackson, J.H. (1878): On affections of speech from disease of the brain. *Brain* **1**, 304–320.

Jacobsen, C.F. (1935): Functions of frontal association areas in primates. *Arch. Neurol. Psychiat.* **33**, 558–569.

Jastrowitz, M. (1888): Localisation im Grosshirn und ueber deren praktische Verwerthung. *Deutsche medizinische Wochenschrift* **14**, 81–83, 108–112, 125–128, 151–153, 172–175, 188–192, 209–211.

Kennard, M.A. (1938): Reorganization of motor function in the cerebral cortex of monkeys deprived of motor and premotor areas in infancy. *J. Neurophysiol.* **1**, 477–497.

Kennard, M.A. (1940): Relation of age to motor impairment in man and subhuman primates. *Arch. Neurol. Psychiat.* **44**, 377–397.

Kleist, K. (1923): *Kriegsverletzungen des Gehirns in ihre Bedeutung fuer die Hirnlokalisation und Hirnpathologie*. Leipzig: Barth.

Kleist, K. (1934): *Gehirnpathologie*. Leipzig: Barth

Levin, H.S., Ewing-Cobbs, L. & Benton, A.L. (1984): Age and recovery from brain damage. In: *Aging and recovery of function in the central nervous system*, ed. S.W. Scheff. New York: Plenum.

Liepmann, A. (1900): Das Krankheitsbild der Apraxie (motorische Asymbolie). *Monatsschrift Psychiatr. Neurol.* **8**, 15–44, 102–132, 182–197.

Marie, P. (1906): Révision de la question de l'aphasie: la troisième circonvolution frontale gauche ne joue aucun rôle dans la fonction du langage. *Semaine médicale* **26**, 241–247.

McFie, J., Piercy, M.F. & Zangwill, O.L. (1950): Visual-spatial agnosia associated with lesions of the right cerebral hemisphere. *Brain* **73**, 167–190.

Nadeau, S. & Crosson, B. (1995): A guide to the functional imaging of cognitive processes. *Neuropsychiat. Neuropsychol. Behav. Neurol.* **8**, 143–162.

Nielsen, J.M. (1936): *Agnosia, apraxia, aphasia: their value in cerebral localization*. New York: Paul B. Hoeber.

Oppenheim, H. (1890): Zur Pathologie der Gehirngeschwuelste. *Arch. Psychiatr.* **21**, 560–578, 705–745. **22**, 27–72.

Orton, S.T. (1925): 'Word-blindness' in school children. *Arch. Neurol. Psychiat.* **14**, 581–615.

Pizzamiglio, L., DePascali, C. & Vignati, A. (1974): Stability of dichotic listening test. *Cortex* **10**, 203–205.

Rieger, C. (1909): Ueber Apparate in dem Hirn. *Arbeiten aus der Psychiatrischen Klinik Wuerzburg* **5**, 176–192.

Russell, W.R. & Espir, M.L.E. (1961): *Traumatic aphasia*. Oxford & London: Oxford University Press.

Schiller, F. (1965): The rise of the 'enteroid process' in the 19th century. *Bull. Hist. Med.* **39,** 326–338.

Scoville, W.B. & Milner, B. (1957): Loss of recent memory after bilateral hippocampal lesions. *J. Neurol. Neurosurg. Psychiat.* **20,** 11–21.

Spreen, O., Risser, A.H. & Edgell, D. (1995): *Developmental neuropsychology*, 2nd edn. New York: Oxford University Press.

St. James Roberts, I. (1979): Neurological plasticity, recovery from brain insult and child development. *Adv. Child Dev. Behav.* **14,** 253–319.

Telfer, W. (1955): *Cyril of Jerusalem and Nemesius of Emesa*. Philadelphia: Westminster Press.

Turkewitz, G. & Ross, P. (1983): Changes in visual field advantage for facial recognition. *Cortex* **19,** 179–185.

Valenstein, E.S. (1986): *Great and desperate cures*. New York: Basic Books.

Vignolo, L.A. (1988): The anatomical and pathological basis of aphasia. In: *Aphasia*, eds. F.C. Rose, R. Whurr & M.A. Wyke. London: Ond Whurr Publishers.

Vincent, C. (1936): Neurochirurgische Betrachtungen ueber die Funktionen des Frontallappens. *Deutsche Med. Wochenschrift* **62,** 41–45.

Welt, L. (1888): Ueber Charakterveraenderungen des Menschen infolge von Laesionen des Stirnhirns. *Deutsche Archiv Klin. Med.* **42,** 339–390.

Chapter 2

The organization of memory in temporo-mesial structures in developmental age

Daria Riva, Veronica Saletti and Francesca Nichelli

Divisione di Neurologia dello Sviluppo, Istituto Nazionale Neurologico Carlo Besta, Via Celoria 11, 20133 Milan, Italy

Summary

Temporo-mesial structures are critical for the organization of long term declarative memories also in developmental age. This means that the architecture of the anatomical structures is established very early in life. Very early lesions can cause memory deficits of different severity and typology and are age-related. Very early lesions (particularly of the hippocampus) irreversibly compromise the capacity to acquire complex modalities of verbal and social communication and to organize a personal and unique cognitive map. Later lesions cause amnesia of different severity, with impairment of episodic memory and preservation of semantic memory if the lesion is localized to the hippocampus, or the impairment of both types of memory in case of hippocampus and parahippocampus localization.

A large number of experimental and clinical studies have demonstrated that temporo-mesial structures play a fundamental role in the organization of memory. The clinical studies have been based on descriptions of patients suffering from global amnesia after undergoing surgery for bilateral temporo-mesial lesions or patients with more selective partial verbal and non-verbal memory deficits due to either left or right unilateral surgical lesions (Frisk & Milner, 1990; Jones-Gotman, 1986; Jones-Gotman *et al.*, 1997; Press *et al.*, 1989; Rausch & Babb, 1993).

More particularly, the temporo-mesial structures are critical for the development of long-term declaratory memories.

The enormous flow of studies in this field began in 1957 with Scoville and Milner's original description of what has now become the historical case of HM, because it has since been the subject of further studies by Milner and other authors (Scoville & Milner, 1957; Corkin, 1984; Milner *et al.*, 1968; Gabrieli *et al.*, 1988). HM underwent bilateral ablation of the temporo-mesial structures because of intractable epilepsy The intervention caused severe anterograde tasks administered in tactile and visual form to children with complete ACC in order to verify whether or not their brain specialization develops normally.

Patients

The study subjects were selected from a larger group of children with ACC on the basis of the following criteria:

(1) Age > 8 years;

(2) Complete CC agenesis documented by CT and MRI;

(3) Normal WISC verbal and performance IQ (Wechsler, 1986);

(4) Absence of severe epilepsy (fewer than five seizures in the two years preceding the evaluation);

(5) Ability to understand the dichotomic procedures;

(6) Consent to participate in the study.

The final sample consisted of the five right-handed children listed in Table 1: all of them had complete agenesis of the corpus callosum. In three cases, other cerebral malformations associated with the agenesis were trigonocephaly (No. 1), a right intraventricular cyst (No. 3) and ventricular malformation (No. 4). Nos. 2, 3 and 5 had experienced slight neonatal asphyxia; the other two children had not had any perinatal problems.

Epilepsy was present in children Nos. 1, 3 and 5, but only No. 5 presented rare complex partial seizures at the time of the tests: No. 1 was receiving carbamazepine anti-epileptic treatment, No. 3 carbamazepine and diazepam, and No. 5 primidone and clobazam. Patient No. 2 had discontinued antiepileptic therapy four years before.

None of them presented any neurological deficit.

Table 1. Demographic, clinical and radiological findings

	Sex	Age	Corpus callosum + other malformations	Anterior commissure	Perinatal asphyxia	Epilepsy
1	F	11.4	CA + trigonocephaly	not visible	no	previous partial
2	M	11.5	CA + slight cortical atrophy	small	slight	no
3	M	14.4	CA + intraventricular cyst	small	slight	previous partial
4	F	15.4	CA + ventricular malformation	not visible	no	no
5	M	9.3	CA	small	slight	present partial

CA = Complete agenesis.

Chapter 3   Hemispheric specialization in acallosal children

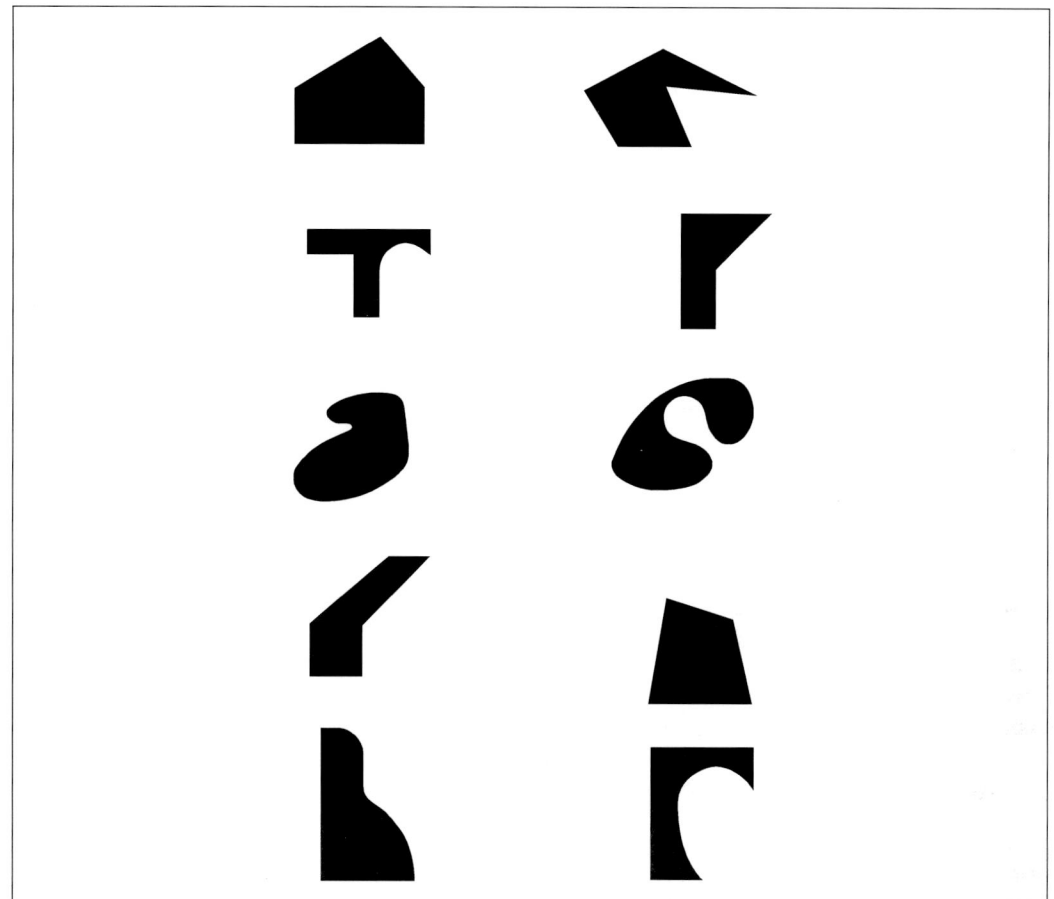

Fig. 1. Non-verbalizable shapes used in dichaptic tactile tasks.

Methods

Dichotomic procedures

Dichaptic tactile procedures

The dichaptic procedures consisted of the blind handling of verbal and non-verbal material for 5 s. Given that the representation of the hands is only contralateral, whereas that of the proximal part of the arms is both homo- and contralateral (Kuypers, 1981), the wrists of the subjects were immobilized in such a way as to allow only manual manipulation.

The verbal material consisted of five pairs of single letters (P–V; H–Z; L–T; I–O; E–A), which were simultaneously and alternately manipulated with the right and left hand.

The non-verbal material consisted of the non-verbalizable shapes illustrated in Fig. 1, which were manipulated in the same way as the letters.

The task was to identify the stimulus manipulated by each hand from a display showing the different letters or shapes. Each stimulus was presented three times in a random manner.

Tachistoscopic procedures

Both verbal and non-verbal material was projected.

Three sets of verbal material were flashed to the right (RVH) and left visual hemifield (LVH): single letters, two-letter patterns and common two-syllable Italian words. Each stimulus was presented for 150 ms with a 3-s interval between stimuli. The total number of stimuli was 60 per hemifield (Riva et al., 1993).

The spatial stimuli were displayed using a 3 x 3 square matrix, with a dot randomly occupying one of the nine possible positions. The square was presented to the RVH and LVH for 100 ms. After a 3-s interval, the answer card with the nine possible positions indicated by a number was displayed in the centre of the screen. The subjects were told in advance that they would be asked to report the location of the dot by naming the corresponding number on the answer card. The total number of stimuli was 27 per hemifield (Riva et al., 1993).

Apparatus

The size of the white cards (trimmed to be used with a G 1128) was 10.2 x 15.2 cm. They were presented using a semi-automatic changer connected with one field of the three-field tachistoscope (model T–3A, G 1128 Gerbrands). The latter was connected to a lamp driver that controlled the switching on of the constant-intensity lights in the fields, as well as to a device for initiating the stimulus that consisted of a digital millisecond timer plus logic interface.

Controls

Five age-matched children with the same number of years of schooling were chosen as controls. Their WISC scores were comparable with those of the studied subjects.

Statistical analysis

The scores obtained using the right and left hand during the manipulation tests, and those obtained from the two hemifields during the tachistoscopic tests, were analysed by means of Student's t-test (two-tailed).

Results

ACC subjects

The tachistoscopic tests revealed that the ACC subjects showed no significant prevalence of either of the two hemifields/hemispheres during both the verbal and spatial localization tests; nor did they show any prevalence during the dichaptic manipulation tests of either the verbal or non-verbal material (Table 2).

Normal subjects

The tachistoscopic tests revealed that the controls showed a significant prevalence of the right visual hemifield/left hemisphere during the verbal tests ($P < 0.01$), and of the left visual hemifield/right hemisphere during the spatial localization tests ($P < 0.1$) (Table 3).

The dichaptic manipulation tests showed that they recognized the letters significantly better with their right hands/left hemisphere ($P < 0.001$), and the non-verbalisable shapes with their left hands/right hemisphere ($P < 0.1$) (Table 3).

Table 2. ACC subjects: WISC data and errors on dichotomic tasks

No.	VIQ	PIQ	Dichaptic tasks				Tachistoscopic tasks			
			Letters/30		Shape/30		Verbal/60		Spatial/60	
			hand		hand		visual field		visual field	
			R	L	R	L	R	L	R	L
1	124	130	2	3	3	3	9	8	1	2
2	117	98	1	2	4	5	7	5	5	2
3	108	97	1	2	6	7	24	24	5	5
4	113	99	3	2	3	4	20	19	10	12
5	126	120	2	1	1	2	3	2	15	15
	TOTAL		9	10	17	21	63	58	36	36
	P		ns		ns		ns		ns	

Table 3. Controls: WISC data and errors on dichotomic tasks

No.	VIQ	PIQ	Dichaptic tasks				Tachistoscopic tasks			
			Letters/30		Shape/30		Verbal/60		Spatial/60	
			hand		hand		visual field		visual field	
			R	L	R	L	R	L	R	L
1	110	132	0	2	1	1	0	2	2	0
2	100	111	0	1	2	0	0	1	2	0
3	124	97	0	2	3	0	1	3	4	1
4	112	103	0	2	3	1	1	4	3	0
5	121	122	0	1	2	0	0	3	2	0
	TOTAL		0	8	11	2	2	13	13	1
	P		< 0.001		< 0.01		< 0.01		< 0.01	

Discussion

Our results can be summarized as follows: the normal subjects showed the usual pattern of hemispherical functional asymmetry (i.e. the prevalence of the left hemisphere for verbal tasks, and that of the right for non-verbal tasks); this pattern was the same whether the tests were administered in a visual or tactile manner.

The functioning of the ACC subjects proved to be more or less symmetrical during all of the tests, without any significant behavioural differences between the left and right hemispheres. Nevertheless, the performances of all of them were characterized by a large number of errors.

These results show a duplication of the abilities necessary to complete the tests used in this study. A large number of studies of acallosal subjects have been carried out, but their results are discordant; however, the majority were concerned with investigating language or language-related abilities, and there are hardly any concerning non-verbal abilities (Meerwarldt, 1993).

Some of these studies have shown that these subjects have a bilateral representation of language (Sperry, 1974; Bryden, 1970; Saul & Gott, 1976; Denenberg, 1981; Ferriss & Dorson, 1975), and these results have been confirmed by Dennis (1976, 1981), who found duplicated hemispherical specialization.

These findings fit well with Cook's (1984, 1986) 'diffuse inhibitory hypothesis', according to which the presence of the corpus callosum does not mean an absence of information in the inhibited regions, but a difference in the activity of the two hemispheres: a specific activity is concentrated in one hemisphere and inhibited in its contralateral counterpart.

Callosal connectivity may differ intra-individually and can be modulated by environmental conditions (Cook, 1986; Kimura, 1967), the conclusion being that callosal connections prevent the bilateralization and duplication of information, and also allow the amplification of subtle informative elements and processing differences between the two hemispheres that are initially due to inherited biological differences.

However, the results of other studies contradict these conclusions (Jeeves, 1986; Lassonde et al., 1981; Lassonde et al., 1986) insofar as they have failed to find any evidence indicating that the CC is necessary to ensure the definitive development of hemispheric specialization. These results return to the concept that, although not explicit and complete at birth, hemispherical specialization is innate and responds to a genetic programme that by definition cannot be changed.

This view is supported by the results of anatomical asymmetry (Chi et al., 1977; Chiarello, 1980; Galaburda et al., 1978), and even prenatal neurofunctional studies (Barnet et al., 1974; Berlin & McNeil, 1976; Caplan & Kinsbourne, 1976); Witelson (1985a) also maintains that the CC is not necessary for the development of hemispherical specialization but, at most, it may contribute to its maintenance (Kinsbourne & Hiscock, 1977).

An increase of the number of lateralized tasks does not mean an increase in hemispheric specialization, but rather an increase in cognition and the consequent presence of more cognition available to be lateralized (Witelson, 1985a). A number of investigators (Flannery & Balling, 1979; Fox et al., 1980; Hiscock & Kinsbourne, 1978; Hynd & Obrzut, 1977; Piazza, 1977) have found no age-related changes in cerebral asymmetry, although this is challenged by Jernigan's recent findings of post-natal changes in brain morphology (Jernigan & Tallal, 1990).

Finally, Lassonde et al. (1981, 1986, 1988) have described a new pattern of specialization in acallosals: i.e. the prevalence of the right hemisphere over both verbal and non-verbal material. These results, which Lassonde interprets as functional reorganization, can also be explained within the terms of the model described by Goldberg & Costa (1981), according to which the right hemisphere is superior to the left during the initial phases of the acquisition of any kind of skill, with the left hemisphere coming into play only when its greater ability to handle routine and automatic codes becomes more important. This would therefore indicate a shift from the right to the left hemisphere whenever automatic processing is required (Bradshaw & Gates, 1978; Gordon & Carmon, 1976; Hellige, 1976; Reynolds & Jeeves, 1977). In the absence of a corpus callosum, this could lead to the persistence of the immature configuration of the prevalence of the right hemisphere and a failure to evolve towards the superiority of the left hemisphere in the performance of verbal tasks, as suggested by Lassonde's results.

A view encompassing these different positions would not be incompatible with a genetic programme that establishes specialization in an *a priori* manner, as well as the variables related to the morphological development of different brain areas including the CC (Yakovlev & Lecours, 1967).

Although each hemisphere is capable of processing the functions for which it is not strictly competent, the specialized hemisphere performs 'its' functions in a more sophisticated, efficient and rapid manner. When freed of the inhibitory influence of their contralateral, both the left and the right hemisphere are capable of carrying out their specific functions (Gazzaniga, 1970; Gazzaniga & Hillyard,1971).

Our results not only demonstrate symmetrical performance in ACC subjects, but the higher number of errors in comparison with controls (despite the fact that their cognitive capacities were within the normal range) confirms the fact that hemispherical duplication reduces efficiency.

Some authors have maintained that, although the CC can temporarily act as an inhibitor of the establishment of hemispherical specialization (Selnes, 1974), once specialization has been established, this inhibition is no longer necessary and the main function of the CC in adult life is to transfer information from one hemisphere to the other. However, isolated studies of surgical patients have shown that a lesioned CC is capable of modifying the superiority of the left hemisphere in verbal tests even in adults (Leiguarda *et al.*, 1989).

Our results indicate a duplication of the examined functions, not necessarily for all possible tests, but certainly for the tests used in this study.

Compensatory mechanisms in the case of CC agenesis still have to be discussed. These include: (1) behavioural cross-cueing strategies (Gazzaniga, 1970); (2) the bilateral representation of functions (Ferriss & Dorson, 1975; Sperry, 1974); (3) the increased use of ipsilateral pathways (Dennis, 1976; Reynolds & Jeeves, 1977); and (4) the increased use of the extra-callosal commissures (Ettlinger *et al.*, 1972, 1974).

In his review of these mechanisms, Chiarello (1980) claims the priority of the use of other commissures, but does not exclude multiple compensation.

The use of cross-cueing strategies seems to be highly unlikely in the case of dichotomous and particularly tachistoscopic tests. Furthermore, their use should lead to a progressive improvement in performance over time, but this is contradicted by the stable functioning pattern of these subjects.

Increased reliance on ipsilateral pathways may apply in the case of motor or sensory functions but, in this study, the subjects were obliged to use only the distal movements mediated by crossed pathways, because the immobilization of their wrists made it impossible for them to use ipsilateral pathways for proximal movements (Kuypers, 1981). As far as lateralized visual stimuli are concerned, ipsilateral pathways do not exist (Fischer *et al.*, 1992; Chiarello, 1980).

In our opinion, the duplication of hemispheric competences is not a separate mechanism from the use of alternative commissures, particularly the anterior commissure. Dual representation is supported by the results of dichotic studies and the absence of anomia for the stimuli presented in the left visual hemifield; in only one ACC case with bilateral language representation documented by the use of sodium amytal has a precise description been given of the extra-callosal commissures (Fischer *et al.*, 1992; Saul & Gott, 1976).

The degree of hemispheric specialization correlates with the size of the CC (Berrebi *et al.*, 1988;

De LaCoste-Utamsing & Holloway, 1982; Witelson, 1985a, which is known to vary considerably from person to person (Sperry, 1968; Greenblatt, 1983), but also with the considerable difference in the subcortical commissures (Fischer et al., 1992; Saul & Gott, 1976) of normal and ACC subjects, particularly the anterior commissure (Jeeves, 1990). In ACC subjects, the subcortical commissures play an important role in the transfer of information between the two hemispheres, but they may also play an equally important role in determining hemispheric specialization.

This may possibly explain the discordant results of the studies involving ACC subjects: well-represented paleocortical commissures may assure normal specialization, whereas their under-representation may lead to a duplication in hemispheric abilities or an even more immature pattern such as that described by Lassonde (1981, 1984). Furthermore, the studies carried out in this area never report the results of a radiological examination of the commissures (or at least of the anterior commissure), and therefore it is not possible to make a correlation between test results and this type of morphological data.

The MRI examinations of our subjects were not intended to study the paleocortical commissures, but all of the scans were retrospectively reviewed in an attempt to identify at least the anterior commissure: this was not visible in Nos. 1 and 4, and was very small in the other three patients. Although these findings need to be interpreted with extreme caution, they seem to validate our findings of a duplication of the studied functions because the smallness of the anterior commissure would have prevented the development of normal hemispheric specialization (Fischer et al., 1992; Saul & Gott, 1976).

Longitudinal studies of children are necessary in order to establish the role of the corpus callosum towards determining hemispheric specialization. Studies of the anterior and posterior subcortical commissures are also of fundamental importance because their compensatory function in ACC subjects may be complete or partial, and thus lead to the apparently conflicting results of the studies of children in this field.

In this sense, the good compensation described by Lassonde (1981,1984) in children undergoing early callosotomy, in comparison with that observed in those undergoing later surgery, highlights the importance of the institution of alternative pathways such as the paleocommissures, particularly if it takes place at an early age. The establishment of hemispheric specialization even in the absence of a corpus callosum goes in the same direction: the role of the paleocommissures is crucial because they may be considerably reinforced. This developmental adaptation, which is also affected by environmental stimulation, could be additional to what are known to be large and natural interindividual differences in size. Consequently, the establishment of hemispheric functional asymmetry may vary from a high degree of specialization to the duplication of the processing of the various functions.

References

Barnet, A.B., Sotillo, M. & Campos, M. (1974): EEG sensory evoked potentials in early infancy malnutrition, Paper presented to the Society for Neuroscience, St Louis.

Berlin, C.I. & McNeil, M.R. (1976): Dichotic listening. In: *Contemporary issues in experimental phonetics*, ed. N.J. Lass. New York: Academic Press.

Berrebi, A.S., Fitch, R.H., Ralphe, D.L., Deneberg, J.O., Friedrich, Jr, J.L. & Denenberg, V.H. (1988): Corpus callosum: region-specific effects of sex, early experience and age. *Brain Res.* **438**, 216–224.

Bradshaw, J.L. & Gates, E.A. (1978): Visual field differences in verbal tasks: effects of task familiarity and sex of subject. *Brain Lang.* **5,** 166–187.

Bryden, M.P. (1970): Laterality effects in dichotic listening: relations with handedness and reading ability in children. *Neuropsychologia* **8,** 443–450.

Caplan, P.J. & Kinsbourne, M. (1976): Baby drops the rattle, asymmetry in duration of grasp by infants. *Child Dev.* **47,** 532–534.

Chi, J.G., Dooling, E.C. & Gilles, F.H. (1977): Left-right asymmetries of the temporal speech areas of the human fetus. *Arch. Neurol.* **34,** 346–348.

Chiarello, C. (1980): A house divided? Cognitive functioning with callosal agenesis. *Brain Lang.* **2,** 128–158.

Cook, N.D. (1984): Callosal inhibition: the key to the brain code. *Behav. Sci.* **26,** 235–255.

Cook, N.D. (1986): *The brain code. Mechanisms of information transfer and the role of the corpus callosum*, p. 255. London: Methuen.

De LaCoste-Utamsing, M.C. & Holloway, R.L. (1982): Sexual dimorphism in the human corpus callosum. *Science* **216,** 1431–1432.

Denenberg, V.H. (1981): Hemispheric laterality in animals and the effects of early experience. *Behav. Brain. Sci.* **2,** 1–49.

Dennis, M. (1976): Impaired sensory and motor differentiation with corpus callosum agenesis: a lack of callosal inhibition during ontogeny? *Neuropsychologia* **14,** 455–469.

Dennis, M. (1981): Language in congenitally acallosal brain. *Brain Lang.* **12,** 33–53.

Elberger, A.J. (1986): The role of the corpus callosum in visual development. In: *Two hemispheres-one brain. Functions of the corpus callosum*, eds. F. Leporé, M. Ptito & H.H. Jasper, pp. 281–298. New York: Alan R Liss.

Ettlinger, G., Blakemore, C.B., Milner, A.D. & Wilson, J. (1972): Agenesis of the corpus callosum: a behavioral investigation. *Brain* **95,** 327–346.

Ettlinger, G., Blakemore, C.B., Milner, A.D. & Wilson, J. (1974): Agenesis of the corpus callosum: a further behavioral investigation. *Brain* **97,** 225–234.

Ferriss, G.S. & Dorson, M.M. (1975): Agenesis of the corpus callosum: neuropsychological studies. *Cortex* **2,** 95–122.

Fischer, M., Ryan S.B. & Dobyns, W.B. (1992): Mechanisms of interhemispheric transfer and patterns of cognitive function in acallosal patients of normal intelligence. *Arch. Neurol.* **49,** 271–277.

Flannery, R.C. & Balling, J.D. (1979): Developmental changes in hemispheric specialization for tactile spatial ability. *Dev. Psychol.* **15,** 364–372.

Fox, R., Axil, R.N., Shea, S.L. & Dumais, S. (1980): Stereopsis in human infants. *Science* **207,** 323–324.

Galaburda, A.M., LeMay, M., Kemper, T.K. & Geschwind, N. (1978): Right-left asymmetries in the brain. *Science* **199,** 852–856.

Gazzaniga, M.S. (1970): *The bisected brain*, pp. 172. New York: Appleton Century Croft.

Gazzaniga, M.S. & Hillyard, S.A. (1971): Language and speech capacity of the right hemisphere. *Neuropsychologia* **9,** 273–280.

Goldberg, E. & Costa, L. (1981): Hemispheric differences in the acquisition and use of descriptive systems. *Brain Lang.* **14,** 144–173.

Gordon, H.W. & Carmon, A. (1976): Transfer of dominance in speed of verbal response to visually presented stimuli from right to left hemisphere. *Percept. Motor Skills* **42,** 1091–1100.

Greenblatt, S.H. (1983): Localization of the lesions in alexia. In: *Localization in neuropsychology*, ed. A. Kertesz, pp. 324–356. New York: Academic Press.

Hellige, J.B. (1976): Changes in same-different laterality patterns as a function of practice and stimulus quality. *Percept. Psychophys.* **20,** 267–273.

Hiscock, M. & Kinsbourne, M. (1978): Ontogeny of cerebral dominance: evidence from time sharing asymmetry in children. *Dev. Psychol.* **14,** 321–329.

Hynd, G.W. & Obrzut, J.E. (1977): Effects of grade level and sex on the magnitude of dichotic ear advantage. *Neuropsychologia* **15,** 689–692.

Jeeves, M.A. (1986): Callosal agenesis: neuronal and developmental adaptations. In: *Two hemispheres-one brain. Functions of the corpus callosum,* eds. F. Leporé, M. Ptito & H.H. Jasper, pp. 281–298. New York: Alan R. Liss.

Jeeves, M.A. (1990): Agenesis of the corpus callosum. In: *Handbook of neuropsychology,* vol. 4, eds. F. Boller & J.Grafman, pp. 99–114. Amsterdam: Elsevier Science Publishers.

Jernigan, T.L. & Tallal, P. (1990): Late childhood changes in brain morphology observable with MRI. *Dev. Med. Child Neurol.* **32,** 379–385.

Kimura, D. (1967): Functional asymmetry of the brain in dichotic listening. *Cortex* **3,** 163–178.

Kinsbourne, M. & Hiscock, M. (1977): Does cerebral dominance develop? In: *Language development and neurological theory,* eds. S.J. Segalowitz & F.A. Gruber, pp. 172–193. New York: Academic Press.

Kuypers, H.G.J.M. (1981): Anatomy of the descending pathways. In: *Handbook of physiology, Section I. The nervous system,* ed. J.M. Brookhart, pp. 597–666. Bethesda: American Physiological Society.

Lassonde, M., Lortie, J., Ptito, M. & Geoffroy, G. (1981): Hemispheric asymmetry in callosal agenesias revealed by dichotic listening performance. *Neuropsychologia* **19,** 455–458.

Lassonde, M., Ptito M. & Laurencelle L. (1984): Etude tachistoscopique de la spécialisation hémisphérique chez l'agénesique du corps calleux. *Rev. Canad. Psychologie* **38,** 527–536.

Lassonde, M., Sauerwein, H., Geoffroy, G. & Decarie M. (1986): Effects of early and late transection of the corpus callosum in children. A study of tactile and tactuomotor transfer and integration. *Brain* **109,** 953–967.

Lassonde, M., Sauerwein, H., McGabe, N., Laurencelle, L. & Geoffroy, G. (1988): Extent and limits of cerebral adjustment to early section or congenital absence of the corpus callosum. *Behav. Brain Res.* **30,** 165–183.

Leiguarda, R., Starkstein, S. & Berthier, M. (1989): Anterior callosal haemorrhage: a partial interhemispheric disconnection syndrome. *Brain* **112,** 1019–1037.

Meerwarldt, J.D. (1993): Disturbances of spatial perception in a patient with agenesis of the corpus callosum. *Neuropsychologia* **21,** 161–165.

Milner, A.D. & Jeeves, M.A. (1979): A review of behavioural studies of agenesis of the corpus callosum. In: *Structure and function of the cerebral commissures,* eds. I.S. Russel, M.W. Hof & G. Berlucchi, pp. 428–448. Baltimore: Univ. Park.

Piazza, P.M. (1977): Cerebral lateralization in young children as measured by dichotic listening and finger tapping tasks. *Neuropsychologia* **15,** 417–425.

Reynolds, Q. & Jeeves, M.A. (1977): Further studies of crossed and uncrossed pathways responding in callosal agenesis – reply to Kinsbourne and Fisher. *Neuropsychologia* **12,** 287–90.

Riva, D., Pantaleoni, C., Milani, N. & Giorgi, C. (1993): Hemispheric specialization in children with unilateral epileptic focus, with and without computed tomography-demonstrated lesion. *Epilepsia* **34,** 69–73.

Saul, R.E. & Gott, P.S. (1976): *Language and speech lateralization by amytal and dichotic listening test in agenesis of the corpus callosum,* vol. 42, pp. 138–141. Los Angeles, California: UCLA Brain Information Service.

Selnes, O.A. (1974): The corpus callosum. Some anatomical and functional considerations with special reference to language. *Brain Lang.* **1,** 3–39.

Sperry, R.W. (1968): Plasticity of neural maturation, *Dev. Biol.* (**Suppl. 2**), 306–327.

Sperry, R.W. (1970): Perception in the absence of the neocortical commissures. *Res. Publ. Ass. Res. Nerv. Ment. Dis.* **48,** 123–138.

Sperry, R.W. (1974): Lateral specialization in the surgically separated hemispheres. In: *The neuroscience,* eds. F.O. Schmitt & F.G. Worden, pp. 5–19. Cambridge, Mass.: MIT Press.

Wechsler, D. (1986): *Wisc-R. Scala di Intelligenza Wechsler per Bambini Riveduta*. Firenze: Organizzazioni Speciali.

Witelson, S.F. (1985a): On hemisphere specialization and cerebral plasticity from birth: Mark II. In: *Hemisphere function and collaboration in the child*, ed. C.T. Best, pp. 33–85. Orlando: Academic Press Inc.

Witelson, S.F. (1985b): The brain connection: the corpus callosum is larger in left-handers. *Science* **229**, 665–668.

Yakovlev, P.I. & Lecours, A. (1967): The myelogenetic cycles of regional maturation of the brain. In: *Regional development of the brain in early life*, ed. A. Minkovski, pp. 3–65. Oxford: Blackwell.

Chapter 4

Interhemispheric communication in children with callosal agenesis

Daniela Brizzolara and Paola Brovedani

Divisione di Neuropsichiatria Infantile, Università di Pisa, Istituto Scientifico Stella Maris, via dei Giacinti 2, 56018 Calambrone, Pisa, Italy

Summary

Callosal agenesis patients without associated central nervous system abnormalities, which frequently accompany the congenital absence of the largest and most efficient pathway of communication between the hemispheres, are ideal candidates for verifying the hypothesis that absence or reduction of interhemispheric integration may negatively affect cognitive development. These children generally have below average intelligence, may show subtle neuropsychological deficits and, as recent data have demonstrated, can in fact exhibit some disconnection deficits which have been considered typical of split-brain patients. These include impairments in asynchronous bilateral movements, in transferring the locus of touch and tactuomotor learning. Abnormally long latencies in transferring visuo-motor information in simple reaction time paradigms have been reported in acallosal children. In this paradigm, reaction times to simple visual stimuli presented on the opposite side of the responding hand (crossed condition) are much longer than those elicited by ipsilateral stimuli (uncrossed condition). The CUD (crossed-uncrossed difference) of acallosals (in the order of 20 ms) is much greater than that estimated in normal adults (around 4 ms) and children (from 21 to 2 ms depending on the age of the child and on the methodology used), but nevertheless of smaller magnitude with respect to split-brain patients (around 50 ms). This implies that extra-callosal pathways may compensate the congenital absence of the corpus callosum in visual integration but not with the same functional efficiency. Likely candidates for functional substitution are: enhanced ipsilateral control, a larger anterior commissure and recruitment of mesencephalic commissures. The congenital absence of the corpus callosum in children does not determine the classical and severe disconnection syndrome seen in commissurotomized adults, thus suggesting the great potential for cerebral plasticity and re-organization of the young brain. Compensation is however not complete since deficits in interhemispheric integration in the tactile and tactuo-motor domain have been reported as well as the known increase in interhemispheric transfer time of simple visuo-motor information.

Callosal agenesis

Callosal agenesis is a congenital malformation of midline structures of the brain which may occur in isolation or, more often, associated with other developmental abnormalities, both within the central nervous system and other organ systems. Neuroimaging techniques have recently demonstrated numerous subcortical and cortical abnormalities associated with agenesis of the corpus callosum (ACC) such as gray matter heterotopias (Cioni et al., 1994), polymicrogyrias, limbic abnormalities (Atlas et al., 1986). More than 50 different disorders have been reported to be associated with ACC. Five diseases are most frequently associated with ACC: Andermann, Aicardi, Shapiro, Acrocallosal and Menkes. In a series of 83 agenetic children described by Geoffroy (1994), 50 per cent had definite clinical syndromes, mainly Andermann syndrome (22 per cent). Severe to moderate mental retardation was frequent (22 per cent of the cases), whereas epilepsy affected 19 per cent of the sample.

A high incidence (73–80 per cent) of mental retardation in children with ACC affected by neurological diseases is also reported in a series of 705 cases reviewed by Jeret & co-workers (1987). There are, however, increasing reports of patients with pure callosal agenesis who may be asymptomatic and are ideal candidates to verify the hypothesis that congenital absence or reduction of interhemispheric communication may negatively affect cognitive development (Cook, 1984). Numerous cases of children with ACC have been identified by means of routine pre- and post-natal sonography in neonatal intensive care units (Cioni et al., 1994). Normal intellectual development has been documented in acallosal children and adolescents (Sauerwein et al., 1994; Geffen et al., 1994; Temple & Ilsley, 1994) although in most cases the IQ falls in the low-average range. However, subtle deficits in both verbal and visuospatial cognitive functions have been detected by the studies just mentioned. Acallosal children have proven to have poor phonological skills in tasks such as letter fluency and rhyming detection and in the acquisition of orthographic-phonological correspondences in reading as well as subtle deficits in visuo-constructive tasks, such as jigsaw puzzles and in drawing. Memory problems have been reported for complex visual material (Rey Fig. B) by Temple & Ilsley and by Geffen & co-workers in auditory verbal learning tasks, with poor recall of auditorily presented words. However, in the latter case, MRI showed extra-callosal abnormalities, including the absence of the hippocampal commissures, which could be responsible for the memory deficits.

In their extensive review of cognitive development in ACC, Lassonde et al. (1991) conclude that 'the absence of the corpus callosum may prevent the fine tuning of certain cognitive and motor processes without necessarily affecting the general level of functioning'. They also state that most samples of acallosal subjects studied are biased towards a neurologically-affected population and that there is a need to study cases with normal or superior mental abilities to obtain a clear picture of the role of the CC in cognitive development.

Disconnection syndrome in callosal agenesis: is it there?

Split-brain patients exhibit the dramatic signs of the so-called 'disconnection syndrome'(Gazzaniga,1995), being unable to perform tasks that require interhemispheric integration; for instance, they cannot name objects or read words tachistoscopically presented in the left visual field, projecting to the right hemisphere (hemianomia and hemialexia), in striking contrast with their retained capacity to perform the same tasks when the stimuli are presented in the right visual field, projecting to the left hemisphere (for a more detailed description of the syndrome see the chapter by Tassinari in this volume).

The absence of the 'disconnection syndrome' in children born without the corpus callosum has been a well-established datum until very recently. Michael Gazzaniga, in his classical book 'The bisected brain' (1970), noted that acallosals seem to be capable of interhemispheric integration unlike split-brain patients, probably because they develop behavioural compensatory strategies.

An eleven-year-old acallosal boy tested by Gazzaniga could perfectly name words presented in the left visual field and objects palpated both with the right and the left hand. Other researchers have interpreted the absence of disconnection deficits in acallosals as due to compensatory neural pathways functionally substituting the corpus callosum during development (Lassonde *et al.*, 1991). In this study, intermanual comparison of objects and shapes and intermanual localization of touch was perfectly achieved both in acallosal and in early callosotomized subjects; the lack of impairment in tasks requiring callosal integration has been interpreted by Lassonde and co-workers as due to 'the development, alteration and/or selective reinforcement of connections (ipsilateral or subcortico-cortical) that would not have been formed or reinforced under normal circumstances'. However, very recently (Lassonde *et al.*, 1995), the presence of disconnection symptoms in children with callosal agenesis has been reported, providing evidence for limits to the plasticity of the young brain. Although some of the classical disconnection symptoms, such as hemialexia for written stimuli presented in the left visual field and anomia for objects palpated in the left hand have not been reported in acallosals (Milner & Jeeves, 1979; Sauerwein *et al.*, 1981), evidence for other deficits of interhemispheric integration has been recently produced. Impairments in asynchronous bilateral distal movements have been detected (Silver & Jeeves, 1994) in acallosal children as well as problems in transferring tactuomotor learning (Sauerwein *et al.*, 1994) and in localizing the finger opposite to the stimulated one in the contralateral hand (Geffen *et al.*, 1994).

Deficits in interhemispheric transfer of spatial tactile information in acallosal children have also been found (Meerwaldt, 1983; Jeeves & Silver, 1988). Abnormally long interhemispheric visuomotor transfer times have been estimated in acallosals, although not as long as in split-brain patients (Milner, 1994). We will discuss in some detail the experiments with paradigms requiring visuomotor integration.

Interhemispheric transmission of visuomotor information in callosal agenesis

Measures of interhemispheric transfer time obtained with paradigms requiring motor responses to visual stimuli have been used in acallosal subjects. The rationale behind these experiments is the following: unimanual distal responses to a simple visual stimulus presented on the same side as the responding hand (uncrossed condition) are faster than those made to contralateral stimuli (crossed condition).

Because of the organization of the visual and motor pathways, in the uncrossed condition, the hemisphere that receives stimulation is also the one initiating the motor response, while in the crossed condition information must be transferred from the hemisphere receiving stimulation to the one emitting the response. Interhemispheric transmission, presumably across the corpus callosum, can be estimated by calculating the crossed-uncrossed difference (CUD). The mean CUD of normal adults derived across studies is 3.8 ms (for a meta-analysis see Marzi *et al.*, 1991).

As for the CUD in childhood, estimates of interhemispheric transmission time vary across the few studies in the literature. Jeeves (1972) reports a CUD of 1.8 ms to unpatterned stimuli in 9–11-year-old right handed children; Davidson *et al.* (1990) find a CUD of 2.2 ms to checkerboard stimuli in a group of normal and dyslexic 9–12-year olds. Recently, Brizzolara *et al.* (1994) have found significant decreases of CUD values with age in three groups of children (from 21.5 ms at 7 years of age to 6.6 ms at 11 years). The results, obtained on a large sample of subjects, have been interpreted as reflecting the maturation of the corpus callosum during development (Yakovlev & Lecours, 1967). However, Ratinckx *et al.* (1997) did not find a significant age-related CUD decrease in the range 7 to 11 years. Differences in the experimental apparatus, attentional factors affecting the smallest age group, the presence of negative CUDs may explain differences in findings between the two studies. More data, given also the large variability in CUDs in small children, are necessary to give a strong support to the notion that the speed of interhemispheric transfer of information becomes more efficient with age because of callosal maturation. Acallosals should be impaired in visuo-motor reaction time tasks requiring callosal integration (namely, responding with the hand contralateral to the visual stimulus), but not in tasks that do not require interhemispheric transfer of information (hand and stimulus on the same side). The prediction has been tested with a number of acallosal children and adolescents: a 14-year-old boy in Jeeves (1969), a 16-year-old in Kinsbourne & Fisher (1971), an 8-year-old boy in Clarke & Zaidel (1989), a 10-year-old boy in Di Stefano & Salvadori (1998), a 7-year-old boy in Brovedani *et al.* (1996). More data are available on acallosal adults (Lines, 1984; Milner *et al.*, 1985; Di Stefano *et al.*, 1992; Aglioti *et al.*, 1993; Berlucchi *et al.*, 1995; Tassinari *et al.*, 1994). There is strong agreement among different studies in showing that CUD values are abnormally long in subjects with complete congenital absence of the corpus callosum (in most cases around 20 ms), compared to normal adult subjects, but nevertheless shorter than in complete callosotomy patients (CUD of 83.2 ms reported in patient ME in Tassinari *et al.*, 1994). This implies that extra-callosal pathways may compensate the congenital absence of the corpus callosum in visual integration but not with the same functional efficiency. The enhanced development of ipsilateral cortical pathways, the presence of a larger than normal anterior commissure and the role of mesencephalic commissures have been proposed as candidates for functional substitution of the CC. The evidence available so far does not permit the conclusion that there is a single compensatory mechanism at work. As for interhemispheric transfer of simple visual information there is some evidence that the integration may take place at the level of the subcortical commissures (Sergent, 1990; Milner, 1994); in fact acallosal subjects' CUDs are affected by manipulation of visually coded properties of the stimuli like luminance and eccentricity, while normal subjects' CUDs are not. Bimanual coordination difficulties in acallosal children, on the other hand, would reveal the presence of uncrossed ipsilateral pathways competing with crossed contralateral ones, in the absence of a supposedly inhibitory role of the callosum on the development of the former. The anterior commissure may play a role in interhemispheric transmission of visual information; a recent study of two acallosal boys performing a visuomotor integration task has shown that only the boy lacking the anterior commissure was impaired but not the one sparing it (Lassonde, personal communication).

Conclusions

The few subtle deficits found in children with callosal agenesis are an excellent example of cerebral plasticity and brain reorganization. Although the neuropsychological bases of the neural rearrangement taking place in the early phases of development are not fully understood, some hypotheses have been put forward which await further investigation. The use of functional neuroimaging techniques applied to the study of the acallosal brain may permit a rapid progress in our understanding of the neural basis of the functional substitution in the congenital absence of the corpus callosum.

References

Aglioti, S., Berlucchi, G., Pallini, R., Rossi, G.F. & Tassinari, G. (1993): Hemispheric control of unilateral and bilateral responses to lateralized light stimuli after callosotomy and in callosal agenesis. *Exp. Brain Res.* **95**, 151–165.

Atlas, S.W., Zimmerman, R.A., Bilaniuk, L.T., Rorke, L., Hackney, D.B., Goldberg, H.I. & Grossman, R.I. (1986): Corpus callosum and limbic system: neuroanatomic MR evaluation of developmental anomalies. *Radiology* **160**, 355–362.

Berlucchi, G., Aglioti, S., Marzi, C.A. & Tassinari, G. (1995): Corpus callosum and simple visuomotor integration. *Neuropsychologia* **33**, 923–936.

Brizzolara, D., Ferretti, G., Brovedani, P., Casalini, C. & Sbrana, B. (1994): Is interhemispheric transfer time related to age? A developmental study. *Behav. Brain Res.* **64**, 179–184.

Brovedani, P., Brizzolara, D., Ferretti, G. & Cioni, G. (1996): Interhemispheric integration in partial callosotomy and callosal agenesis: two developmental cases. Poster presented at NATO ASI Workshop on the Corpus Callosum. Il Ciocco, Castelvecchio Pascoli, Italy, September 1996.

Cioni, G., Bartalena, L., Biagioni, E. & Boldrini, A. (1994): Callosal agenesis: postnatal sonographic findings. In: *Callosal agenesis: a natural split brain?*, eds. M. Lassonde & M.A. Jeeves, pp. 69–76. New York: Plenum Press.

Clarke, J.M. & Zaidel, E. (1989): Simple reaction times to lateralized light flashes. Varieties of interhemispheric communication routes. *Brain* **112**, 849–870.

Cook, N.D. (1984): Callosal inhibition: the key to the brain code. *Behav. Sci.* **29**, 98–110.

Davidson, R.J., Leslie, S.C. & Saron, C. (1990): Reaction time measures of interhemispheric transfer time in reading disabled and normal children. *Neuropsychologia* **28**, 471–485.

Di Stefano, M. & Salvadori, C. (1998): Asymmetry of interhemispheric visuomotor integration in callosal agenesis. *NeuroReport* **9**, 1331–1335.

Di Stefano, M., Sauerwein, H.C. & Lassonde, M. (1992): Influence of anatomical factors and spatial compatibility on the stimulus-response relationship in the absence of the corpus callosum. *Neuropsychologia* **30**, 177–185.

Gazzaniga, M.S. (1970): *The bisected brain*. New York: Appleton-Century Croft.

Gazzaniga, M.S. (1995): Principles of human brain organization derived from split brain studies. *Neuron* **14**, 217–228.

Geffen, G.M., Nilsson, J., Simpson, D.A. & Jeeves, M.A. (1994): The development of interhemispheric transfer of tactile information in cases of callosal agenesis. In: *Callosal agenesis: a natural split brain?*, eds. M. Lassonde & M.A. Jeeves, pp. 185–197. New York: Plenum Press.

Geoffroy, G. (1994): Other syndromes frequently associated with callosal agenesis. In: *Callosal agenesis: a natural split brain?*, eds. M. Lassonde & M.A. Jeeves, pp. 55–62. New York: Plenum Press.

Jeeves, M.A. (1969): A comparison of interhemispheric transmission times in acallosals and normals. *Psychon. Sci.* **16**, 245–246.

Jeeves, M.A. (1972): Hemisphere differences in response rates to visual stimuli in children. *Psychon. Sci.* **27**, 201–203.

Jeeves, M.A. & Silver, P.H. (1988): Interhemispheric transfer of spatial tactile information in callosal agenesis and partial commissurotomy. *Cortex* **24**, 601–604.

Jeret, J.S., Serur, D., Wisniewski, K.E. & Lubin, R.A. (1987): Clinicopathological findings associated with agenesis of the corpus callosum. *Brain Dev.* **9**, 255–264.

Kinsbourne, M. & Fisher, M. (1971): Latency of uncrossed and of crossed reaction in callosal agenesis. *Neuropsychologia* **9**, 471–473.

Lassonde, M., Sauerwein, H., Chicoine, A. & Geoffroy, G. (1991): Absence of disconnexion syndrome in callosal agenesis and early callosotomy: brain reorganization or lack of structural specificity during ontogeny? *Neuropsychologia* **29**, 481–495.

Lassonde, M., Sauerwein, H.C. & Lepore, F. (1995): Extent and limits of callosal plasticity: presence of disconnection symptoms in callosal agenesis. *Neuropsychologia* **33**, 989–1007.

Lines, C.R. (1984): Nasotemporal overlap investigated in a case of agenesis of the corpus callosum. *Neuropsychologia* **22**, 85–90.

Marzi, C.A., Bisiacchi, P. & Nicoletti, R. (1991): Is interhemispheric transfer of visuomotor information asymmetric? Evidence from a meta-analysis. *Neuropsychologia* **29**, 1163–1177.

Meerwaldt, J.D. (1983): Disturbances of spatial perception in a patient with agenesis of the corpus callosum. *Neuropsychologia* **21**, 161–165.

Milner, A.D. & Jeeves, M.A., (1979): A review of behavioural studies of agenesis of the corpus callosum. In: *Structure and function of the cerebral commissures*, eds. I.S. Russell, M.W.Van Hof & G. Berlucchi, pp. 482–488. London: Macmillan.

Milner, A.D. (1994): Visual integration in callosal agenesis. In: *Callosal agenesis: a natural split brain?*, eds. M. Lassonde & M.A. Jeeves, pp. 171–183. New York: Plenum Press.

Milner, A.D., Jeeves, M.A., Silver P.H., Lines, C.R. & Wilson, J. (1985): Reaction times to lateralized visual stimuli in callosal agenesis: stimulus and response factors. *Neuropsychologia* **23**, 323–331.

Ratinckx, E., Brysbaert, M. & d'Ydewalle, G. (1997): Age and interhemispheric transfer time: a failure to replicate. *Behav. Brain Res.* **86**, 161–164.

Sauerwein, H.C., Lassonde, M., Cardu, B. & Geoffroy, G. (1981): Interhemispheric integration of sensory and motor functions in agenesis of the corpus callosum. *Neuropsychologia* **19**, 445–454.

Sauerwein, H.C., Nolin, P. & Lassonde, M. (1994): Cognitive functioning in callosal agenesis. In: *Callosal agenesis: a natural split brain?*, eds. M. Lassonde & M.A. Jeeves, pp. 221–233. New York: Plenum Press.

Sergent, J. (1990): Furtive incursions into bicameral minds. Integrative and coordinating role of subcortical structures. *Brain* **113**, 537–568.

Silver, P.H. & Jeeves, M.A. (1994): Motor coordination in callosal agenesis: In: *Callosal agenesis: a natural split brain?*, eds. M. Lassonde & M.A. Jeeves, pp. 207–219. New York: Plenum Press.

Tassinari, G., Aglioti, S., Pallini, R., Berlucchi, G. & Rossi, G.F. (1994): Interhemispheric integration of simple visuomotor responses in patients with partial callosal defects. *Behav. Brain Res.* **64**, 141–149.

Temple, C. & Ilsley, J. (1994): Sounds and shapes: language and spatial cognition in callosal agenesis. In: *Callosal agenesis: a natural split brain?*, eds. M. Lassonde & M.A. Jeeves, pp. 261–273. New York: Plenum Press.

Yakovlev, P.I. & Lecours, A. (1967): The myelogenetic cycles of regional maturation of the brain. In: *Regional development of the brain in early life*, ed. A. Minkowski, pp. 3–65. London: Blackwell.

Chapter 5

Acquired lesions of the corpus callosum

Giancarlo Tassinari

Dipartimento di Scienze Neurologiche e della Visione, Sezione di Fisiologia Umana, Università di Verona, Strada le Grazie 8, 37134 Verona, Italy

Summary

The acquired disconnection of the two hemispheres of the human brain usually follows therapeutic sections of the corpus callosum, aimed at reducing the spreading of otherwise intractable epilepsies. The state of the art of this approach is briefly reviewed. Complete commissurotomy affects cognition, perception, sensori-motor integration and attention. Cognitive capabilities are impaired whenever the perceiving right, non-speaking hemisphere has to rely upon the disconnected left hemisphere for a verbal or praxic response (left hemifield anomia and alexia, left hand anomia and dyspraxia). In such situation, basically the two halves of the external world are perceived separately in the two hemispheres; however, some integration across the midline of form, colour and orientation of stimuli is still possible. A measure of the separation between the two halves of the brain can be obtained in complete callosotomy subjects through crossed manual responses, which are very slow in comparison to uncrossed ones when executed with a distal movement. There is no slowing with bilateral proximal and with axial movements (indicating that these responses do not require callosal integration in normals), as well as in subjects with partial callosal defects (suggesting that both anterior and posterior callosal routes can subserve the integration of speeded crossed responses). Finally, in complete callosotomy a strong rightward bias in the spatial distribution of visual attention may occur in simple tasks of light detection.

Anatomical and historical introduction

The corpus callosum is the largest of the cerebral or telencephalic commissures (the others being the anterior and the hippocampal commissures). It is also the largest fibre tract of the central nervous system, being made up of a few hundred million different size fibres, both myelinated and unmyelinated, which correspond to 2–8 per cent of all cortical neurons. Neurons projecting to, or receiving from the corpus callosum, can be found in all cytoarchitectonic areas of the cortex. The majority of callosal connections interconnect corresponding points of the neocortex of the two hemispheres (homotopic connections). The far less numerous heterotopic callosal connections link up non-corresponding neocortical regions of the two hemispheres which, however, share some functional properties (for instance, visual occipital areas of one hemisphere and visual temporal areas of the other hemisphere, or somatosensory and motor areas).

Due to the fact that the forebrain commissures are a 'bridge' between two substantially symmetric cerebral hemispheres, the idea that they were crucial for conferring unitarity not only to physiological cortical activities on the two sides, but also to mental processes, has always been tempting. In 1889 Gustav Fechner, the founder of psychophysics, hypothesized that each half of a bisected brain would keep its own consciousness (Fechner, 1889). On the other hand, already in 1871 the philosopher von Hartman put forward the still fantastic hypothesis that two men with their brains united by a callosum-like fibre tract would share the same consciousness (Hartman, 1871).

Starting from the end of last century, a number of interhemispheric disconnection syndromes have been described: Freund's (1889) optic aphasia, Déjerine's (1892) alexia without agraphia, and Liepmann's (1900) unilateral apraxia and agraphia. However, they were consequences of cerebral damage involving the corpus callosum more than lesions limited to the corpus callosum. During the whole first half of this century, animal experimental studies did not produce clear results, mainly due to the use of methods that were inadequate to disclose the effects of interhemispheric disconnection. A single, isolated success dates back to Pavlov's school in the 1920s, with the demonstration that it was impossible for a callosotomized dog to transfer from one body side to the other a conditioned salivary response to a tactile stimulus (Bykov & Speranski, 1924). Shortly after, when the technical aid provided by electroencephalography became available, the role of the corpus callosum in the transhemispheric spread of an electrically or chemically induced seizure was revealed (Gozzano, 1935; Moruzzi, 1939), and this result of animal experimentation started a line of research which led to the first attempts of callosal resection in humans. This surgery was performed on patients with drug refractory forms of epilepsy by the surgeon Van Wagenen in US starting from the beginning of the 1940s (Van Wagenen & Herren, 1940). His attempt was mainly based on the clinical observation that unilateral seizures usually do not cause a loss of consciousness and therefore are less severe than bilateral seizures, which often depend on propagation of discharges through the forebrain commissures. The psychologist Akelaitis studied about 30 patients submitted to partial or total callosotomy (with uncertain therapeutic effects), and surprisingly found no defects which could be specifically attributed to the interhemispheric disconnection (Akelaitis, 1944). This result was strongly in favour of holistic and anti-localizationistic theories of those years, which ascribe nervous integration to effects of electrical fields or diffuse projection systems. Lashley (1951) arrived at the point of stating that the only interhemispheric integration performed by the corpus callosum is that of preventing the two hemispheres from falling apart; and McCulloch (1949) rather paradoxically stated that the sole function of the forebrain commissures is that of spreading epileptic seizures from one side of the brain to the other.

The change was due to Roger Sperry, a strong supporter of the functional specificity of neural centres and selectivity of their interconnections, later a winner of the Nobel Prize in 1981. With his student Ronald Myers, he applied to split-brain animals an experimental paradigm that was based on the perceptual equivalence between different sensory channels (Myers & Sperry, 1953). If two different sensory channels are directed to two separated hemispheres, as happens when presenting visual stimuli through either eye following a midsagittal section of the optic chiasm, their interaction can only occur by way of specific connections between the hemispheres. In fact, split-chiasm cats promptly recognize through one eye (and the corresponding ipsilateral hemisphere) stimuli formerly presented to the other eye and hemisphere; but this transfer becomes impossible following the section of the corpus callosum. In the same years, in California where Sperry was working, the neurosurgeons Vogel and Bogen reintroduced cerebral commissurotomy for the treatment of forms of epilepsy resistant to pharmacological therapy (Bogen & Vogel, 1962), and their series of patients was studied by Sperry and Gazzaniga (Gazzaniga et al., 1962; Sperry et al., 1969). However, the surgical commissurotomy for the treatment of epilepsy has never been practiced routinely. It had a revival in the mid-1970s by Wilson in Dartmouth, NH (Wilson et al., 1975), and then spread also outside North America. In Italy, it is now practiced in two centres, one at the University of Ancona (Papo et al., 1997), the other at the Catholic University in Rome (Pallini et al., 1995).

Further information on the topic of this section can be found in Berlucchi & Aglioti (1999).

Clinical series: a brief overview

The causes of acquired disconnection can be grouped into (a) accidental lesions of vascular, tumoural, traumatic or degenerative origin; (b) surgical lesions as a consequence of a transcallosal approach to tumours or cysts of the third ventricle; and (c) therapeutic sections of telencephalic commissures, performed with the aim of reducing the spread of otherwise intractable forms of epilepsy to the whole brain. The last corresponds to the largest group of cases, and the only one including subjects with complete commissurotomies.

At variance with other surgical therapies of epilepsy, where the epileptogenic focus is identified and extirpated, the section of the corpus callosum has the aim of interrupting the propagation of epileptic discharges. Therefore, it applies mainly to cases with secondary generalization, in which the focus is not easy to detect and then its extirpation cannot be applied. A recent study (Carmant & Holmes, 1994) complains that long-term follow-up studies of callosotomized patients are few, and flawed by the lack of accurate seizure counts and assessments of other parameters inherent to the quality of life. However, Nordgren et al. (1991) reported 68 patients of paediatric age, starting from those of Van Wagenen, and found that all together more than three-quarters displayed a reduction of seizures of at least 50 per cent with a follow-up of at least 6 months. According to their overview, the types of seizures which benefit more of this surgery are brief seizures with a sudden fall to the ground, both atonic and consequent to myoclonic jerks, which often occur many times per day and are the most refractory to control with anticonvulsants; but also generalized tonic or tonic–clonic seizures, which often after callosotomy convert to more focal seizures. Substantially similar results have been reported by Cendes et al. (1993) in 34 cases between 2 and 16 years, with an average follow-up of 42 months. An element of caution emerges in this study, since almost half of the cases with a total section show disconnection symptoms such as reduced verbal production, dysarthria and ataxia. Another large series of patients (Fuiks et al., 1991: 80 cases between 4 and 53 years, mean 18.3) has been presented as evidence that sectioning the anterior 80 per cent of the corpus callosum does not produce a significantly better outcome than a two-stages complete section; however, a different study (Reutens et al., 1993: 64 cases between 3 and 47 years, mean 20.0) found a clear improvement after completion of callosotomy following a first section that was limited to the anterior 50–65 per cent; in fact, Oguni et al. (1991: 43 cases between 8 and 60 years, mean 23.5) reported a clear difference between sections of 50 and 65 per cent; yet still others (Mamelak et al., 1993: 15 cases between 9 and 31 years) concluded that the extent of callosotomy is not an important factor on outcome when at least 50–65 per cent of the callosum is divided. No relationship has been found between the intraoperative transformation of general-

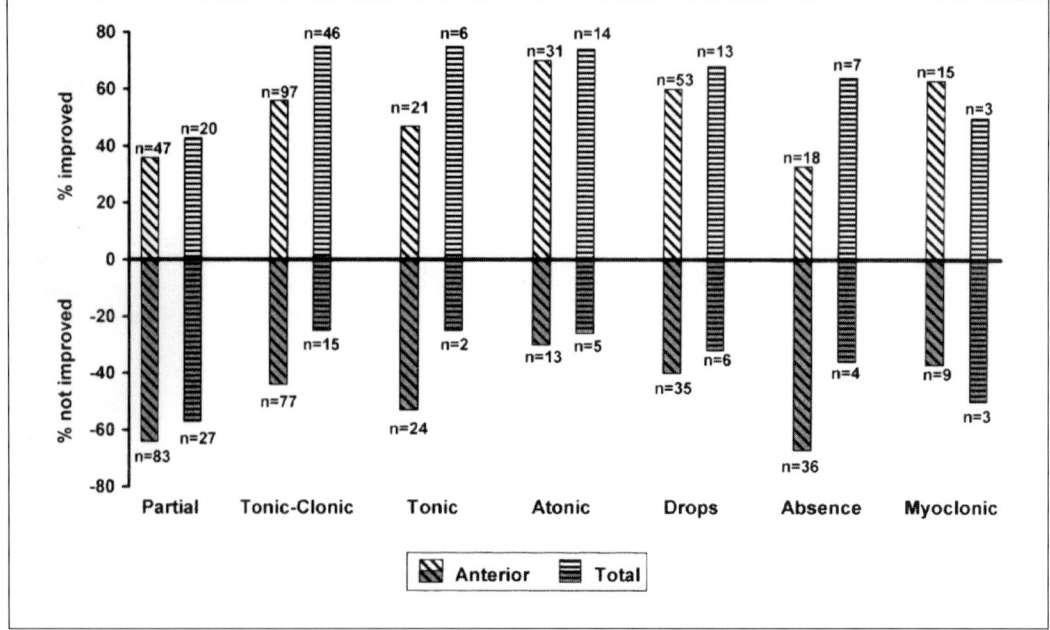

Fig. 1. Comparison of the effects of anterior and total callosotomy on different seizure types in 330 patients (data from Spencer et al., 1993).

ized epileptiform discharges to lateralized activity and the successive control of seizures (Fiol et al., 1993: 37 cases between 3 and 46 years, mean 20.0). Spencer et al. (1993; see Fig. 1), by reviewing a series of overall 330 patients of different ages, concluded that the section of the anterior two thirds of the corpus callosum is effective in the control of atonic seizures, but a complete callosotomy is required for the control of other generalized seizures, mainly of tonic–clonic or tonic type, specially in cases of diffuse cerebral abnormalities (low IQ, polymorphic seizures). Finally, and in agreement with the above study, the study by Papo et al. (1997) reported a series of 36 cases between 14 and 46 years (mean 25.4) and, despite a caution concerning the limited value of factors previously defined as positive (normal IQ, predominance of atonic seizures, anterior EEG foci, abnormal neuromorphological findings) or negative (low IQ, multifocality, polymorphic seizures), concluded that drop-attacks, occurring abruptly, unpreceded by other epileptic features, are definitely better influenced by callosotomy.

Evidence of disconnection in anomia – alexia – apraxia

The semiology of callosal disconnection must start from these striking patterns of separation between the two halves of the brain, which have been studied basically in the adolescent or adult subject.

The seminal studies of Myers & Sperry (1953) in the split-chiasm cat exploited the surgical elimination of the two hemiretinae with a contralateral projection. With an intact visual system, both in normal and disconnected subjects, the stimulation of a single hemisphere must be achieved by limiting visual presentation to the opposite half of the visual field. This is usually obtained by using presentation times that are shorter than those needed to disengage the gaze from the fixation point (tachistoscopic presentation). Longer lateralized presentations are possible, but require different expedients, like asking the subject to keep the gaze at the extreme limits of a lateral fixation, left or right; or 'neutralizing' eye movements by an equivalent, simultaneous displacement of the visual stimulus.

A normal subject has no difficulties in naming simple visual stimuli (colours, pictures of common objects, digits, letters, syllables and words) tachistoscopically presented in either left or right visual hemifield. Instead, patients with a complete interhemispheric disconnection are easily able to name visual stimuli presented in the right, but fail with stimuli presented in the left visual hemifield; however, the same left hemifield stimuli can be recognized in tests of non-verbal identification, and also be associated to objects with similar physical or semantic properties.

A particular case of anomia concerns somatosensory modality. In this case it is easy to separate the afferent channels to the two hemispheres, since it is sufficient to ask the subject to explore objects with either hand. In this case too, the lack of communication between the right hemisphere, where the afferents from the left hand terminate, and the left hemisphere, where the language is located, makes it impossible to name manipulated objects. It is properly a matter of stereognosic anomia of the left hand, which can be confused with a unilateral astereognosis. However, the patient proves not to be agnosic because he is able to retrieve with the left hand in a group of disparate objects the object just manipulated with the same hand.

As for reading, the majority of split-brain patients show in the left hemifield what has been defined by Sugishita *et al.* (1985) 'type I alexia': that is, not only are they unable to read words aloud, but also they fail in understanding words.

Finally, a consequence of disconnection concerning motor control is left hand apraxia, or callosal dyspraxia. The patient is unable to execute with the left hand the gestures which are requested to him verbally; however, he is perfectly able to execute the same gestures with the right hand, or with the left hand itself if he is requested not to execute verbal commands, but to imitate the gestures of an examiner (Fig. 2).

We face here a terminological problem, in the sense that the definition of apraxia implies that the patient should understand the command: which the callosotomized patient is able to do as a whole, but it is his left hemisphere which understands, while it is up to his right hemisphere to execute (in fact, not to execute!) the command. However, the fact that split-brain patients can imitate gestures with the left hand questions another well-established concept of classical neuropsychology, that of a praxic centre lateralized in the dominant left hemisphere (hence the term dyspraxia instead of apraxia).

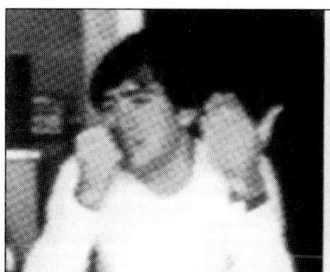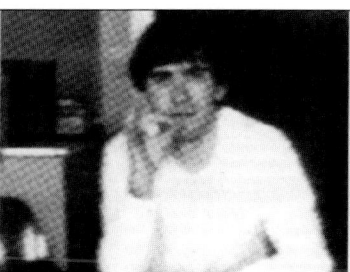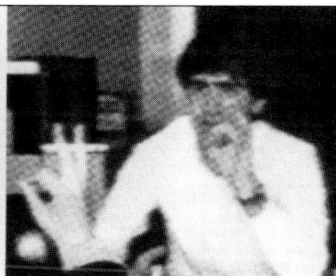

Fig. 2. Callosal dyspraxia in a callosotomized subject. The three photographs from left to right show his failed attempt to make the OK sign on verbal command with the left hand, his successful performance with the right hand, and his equally successful performance when he imitated the examiner with his left hand (modified from Aglioti et al., 1998).

The consequences of early sections of the corpus callosum are more limited than in adulthood: a situation that is somehow comparable to the large compensation in interhemispheric communication taking place in callosal agenesis (Lassonde et al., 1988). Lassonde et al. (1986) compared the performance of five callosotomized children and adolescents between 5 and 16 years in the interhemispheric transfer of tactile information and tactuomotor learning. The younger patients proved to be less affected by callosotomy, possibly because of continued reliance on ipsilateral neural pathways, than the older patients. In turn, ipsilateral pathways could become more effective due to the formation of new connections. More generally, brain reorganization or lack of structural specificity during ontogeny should be taken in account (Lassonde et al., 1991). A similar better outcome for younger children has been recently described by Lassonde & Sauerwein (1997).

Further information on the topic of this section can be found in Berlucchi & Aglioti (1999).

How separated are the two halves? Visual perception across the midline

While initially the research on split-brain patients underlined the independence of the two divided hemispheres, successively many studies have addressed the complementary unitary aspect, which is displayed by patients in everyday life. The experimental approach focused mainly on the integration across the two halves of the visual field. Trevarthen & Sperry (1973) claimed that integration was possible within what they called 'ambient' system, but not within the 'focal' visual system. Focal vision would be cortical, centred in the foveal region and dedicated to detailed vision and object identification; while ambient vision would be subcortical and concerned with space around the body, being more sensitive to visual periphery and to moving stimuli. This distinction had some success, to the point that ambient system has been assimilated to the projections reaching extrastriate visual areas via the superior colliculus and the pulvinar nucleus of the thalamus, which could mediate the 'blind vision' (blindsight) described in lesions of the visual cortex. In the experiments by Trevarthen & Sperry (1973), callosotomized subjects were able to make accurate judgements about the relative motion of large disks and lines presented 45° from fixation in the two hemifields (while being unable to describe their shapes), thus demonstrating interhemispheric transfer within the ambient system. Disconnection was instead evident in focal vision, as shown by studies on the identification of chimeric figures. These comprised half-pictures, like a half-rose and a half-bee, joined at the midline. Each hemisphere seemed to perceive the half contralateral figure as a whole, for instance the patient could verbally report seeing a bee (shown as a half-bee in the right hemifield) while pointing with his left hand to a rose (shown as a half-rose in his left hemifield).

More recent evidence suggests that what matters for interhemispheric transfer of visual information is not the distinction between near and far in relation to the fovea; instead, the simple features of the stimulus, like position and orientation, can be shared by both hemispheres. For instance Holtzman (1984) demonstrated that callosotomized subjects were able to direct their gaze to a specific location in one visual hemifield on the basis of a positional cue briefly flashed in the contralateral hemifield, but only if the cue did not require a discrimination between different forms. The possibility of interhemispheric transfer in split-brain patients was documented further in a series of studies by Sergent (1983, 1986, 1987), who reported that callosotomized subjects could perform a number of tasks requiring integration between the two visual hemifields. They could (a) judge the alignment of, or the angle formed by, two lines presented in the two hemifields, for a very short time and very close to the fixation point, at variance with the stimuli used by Trevarthen & Sperry; (b) decide whether one of a pair of letters presented one on each hemifield was a vowel, or whether one of two colour patches, one in each hemifield, was green; (c) decide whether the total amount of dots flashed across the two hemifields was odd or even, or whether the sum of digits presented on the left and right was greater or less than 10; and finally (d) make quick lexical decisions as whether strings of four letters flashed bilaterally, two per side, were words or non-words.

The above series of successful performances, and specially the last two, seems to be evidence of transfer of high-level information, but also suggests a dissociation between implicit and explicit processing of information, as observed in different forms of agnosia, amnesia, neglect and blindsight. In fact, the subjects can respond rapidly and accurately, but remain unaware of the information upon which their response was based. For instance, they make a correct lexical decision, but fail to read.

However, another possible explanation of the apparent dissociation shown by Sergent has been proposed by Corballis (1994, 1995), who addressed a stringent criticism to Sergent by arguing that the level of accuracy in numeric and lexical decisions she studied could be based upon transfer of merely binary information, like yes/not, or high/low. For instance, in deciding whether the sum of two digits exceeds 10, the transferred information that the digit presented on the left is 'high' or 'low' can be added to the digit read on the right; much in the same way, if any pair of letters could match only with two pairs in the other hemifield, the information about the couple presented on the left can be reduced to 'yes' or 'no' and this would be sufficient for a binary word/non-word decision.

A peculiar aspect of the integration across the visual midline concerns perception of the apparent motion of spatially separated pairs of light, presented one after the other in opposite hemifields. Ramachandran *et al.* (1986) claimed that such a perception is unaffected in the split-brain; subsequently, this result has been substantially confirmed by Corballis (1995), who, however, found a lower resolution in the split-brain as compared with normals: if stimuli were short and their succession was rapid, the callosotomized subject was unable to discriminate successiveness from simultaneity when lights were flashed to opposite hemifields (while correctly judging the succession of two lights in unilateral presentations). Motion detection should be the typical situation involving the subcortical system: area MT, which is crucial for this task in the monkey, receives input from the superior colliculus and the pulvinar nucleus. However, the cortical system seems to be tuned to a higher temporal resolution than the subcortical one. Moreover, the operation of the subcortical system could be limited to detecting temporal succession rather than producing the sensation of continuous displacement which corresponds to the apparent movement *per se*.

How separated are the two halves? The case of the CUD

Poffenberger (1912) showed that the responses of each hand to simple visual stimuli presented on the same side are faster than the responses of the same hand to stimuli presented contralaterally. The advantage (crossed-uncrossed difference or CUD) proves to be between 2 and 6 ms in normal subjects. The simplest explanation of such advantage is offered by neuroanatomy: each hand is controlled by descending pathways from the cortex of the opposite side, which is the same where a visual stimulus ipsilateral to the hand is primarily projected; while responses to contralateral stimuli should require a time-consuming transfer of information from one hemisphere to the other, presumably through the corpus callosum. Theoretical calculations by

Ringo et al. (1994) indicate that the time needed for the transfer through the corpus callosum may vary from less than 5 up to 300 ms; therefore, the CUD of normal subjects should measure the transmission throughout the fastest of callosal fibres. CUD assessment in patients with a complete section of telencephalic commissures led to the conclusion that in the split-brain there is not a total lack of communication between the two hemispheres, in agreement with the observation of a substantial normality of such patients in everyday life. Sergent & Myers (1985), followed by Clarke & Zaidel (1989), and finally Aglioti et al. (1993) showed that in such a situation there is indeed an increase of the CUD, that can reach 50 times the normal value; nevertheless, crossed responses are possible and errorless. It is likely that, in the absence of the corpus callosum, the transmission from one side of the brain to the other takes place between sub-cortical connections. The hippocampal commissure is usually sectioned along with the corpus callosum. The transfer through the anterior commissure can be ruled out since the CUD is not shorter when it is left intact (Aglioti et al., 1993) than when it is severed along with the corpus callosum (Sergent & Myers, 1985; Clarke & Zaidel, 1989). This conclusion is also supported by the long CUDs found in cases where callosal agenesis is associated with a normal or even hyperplastic anterior commissure (Jeeves, 1990; Aglioti et al., 1993).

The Poffenberger paradigm is based on the assumption of a complete crossing of the motor pathways mediating the response. In fact, this assumption is only valid for a limited amount of

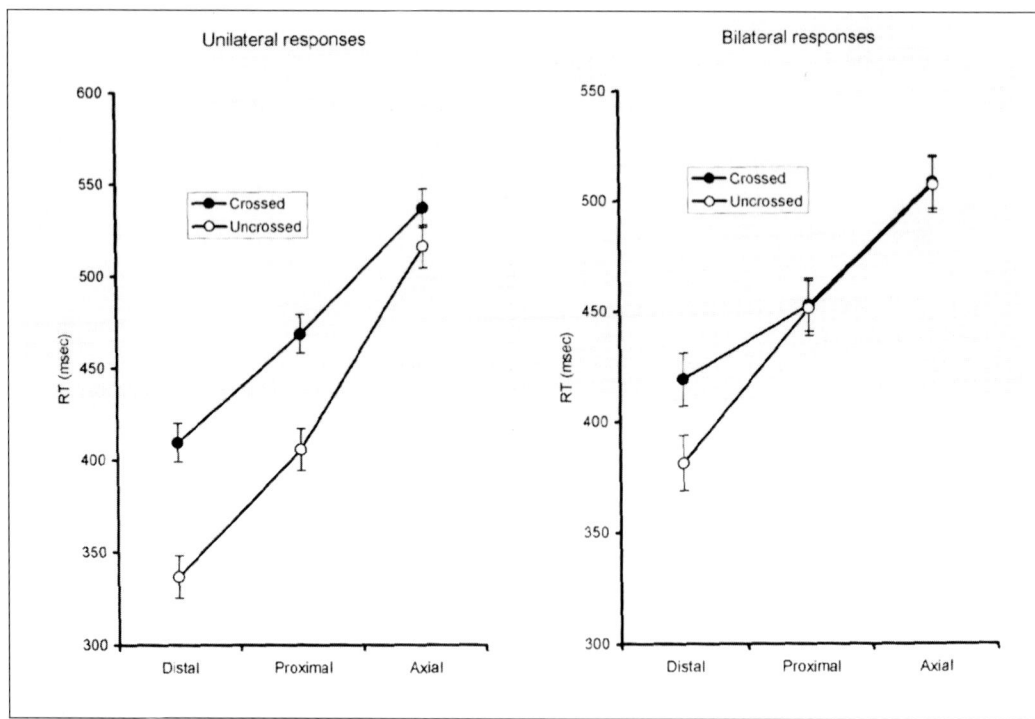

Fig. 3. Reaction time (RT) of a callosotomized subject as a function of different response effectors and unilaterality or bilaterality of response. In the unilateral response condition (left), uncrossed responses are faster than crossed responses with all types of effectors, but the difference is not significant for axial responses. In the bilateral response condition (right), there is a significant difference between crossed and uncrossed RTs in distal, but not in proximal and axial responses (modified from Aglioti et al., 1993).

distal movements, mainly those of single fingers. Axial and proximal muscles involved in global body movements, postural adjustments and integrated limb-body movements are instead under the control of bilaterally distributed motor systems (Kuypers, 1981), so that each hemisphere can activate these muscles on either side without the need of interhemispheric communication. As a consequence, in normal subjects a CUD can be found in the case of distal responses performed both unilaterally and bilaterally, and in proximal responses of flexion of the forearm performed unilaterally, but not in bilateral forearm responses (Di Stefano et al., 1980), nor in axial responses of elevation of the shoulder, either unilateral or bilateral. The results of the split-brain subject clearly confirm the distinction between contralaterally and bilaterally controlled movements. In fact, an enormously increased CUD, due to the interhemispheric disconnection, and to the transfer of information through subcortical connections, is found for distal and unilateral proximal responses (Fig. 3). In the other responses, instead, there is no difference between callosotomized and normal subjects, indicating that bilateral proximal and axial movements are independent from interhemispheric transfer. It is interesting to note that the distinction between unilateral and bilateral control also applies to the facial muscles: when callosotomized subjects are requested to smile, the right side of the mouth starts contracting well before the left side when the command to smile is lateralized to the left; the difference is of the same order as the CUD observed in manual responses of the same subjects. On the contrary, in spontaneous smiling there is no asymmetry between the two sides of the mouth (Gazzaniga & Smylie, 1990).

Acquired lesions of the corpus callosum may help to solve another problem, that of the topography of the interhemispheric transfer. The corpus callosum may subserve the integration of crossed visuomotor reactions by transferring the visual input across the midline, or by transmitting a 'go-signal' to the motor areas of the hemisphere which emits the response (in this case, an intrahemispheric visuomotor transfer should precede the interhemispheric motor transfer). The transfer of sensory information seems unlikely, since the normal CUD remains invariant across major changes in intensity and eccentricity of visual stimuli (Berlucchi et al., 1977), which instead influence the CUD in callosal agenesis (Milner et al., 1985). The alternative hypothesis of a motor transfer is indirectly supported by the finding that the CUD is matched by interhemispheric differences in latencies of potentials evoked by lateralized visual stimuli at central, but not occipital recording sites (Rugg et al., 1984); and by the finding that the CUD is prolonged in frontal or parietal, but not occipital lesions (Anzola & Vignolo, 1992). We measured the CUD using distal responses in seven patients with an anterior (or anterior and middle) section of the corpus callosum, sparing the splenium in each case (Tassinari et al., 1994). There was no evidence of disconnection symptoms, like left alexia, anomia or apraxia, in any of these subjects. Finding a prolonged CUD would have been in favour of the 'motor' transfer, and would have proven that a specific contingent of callosal fibres mediates crossed responses. In fact, our findings did not support this expectation, since in all cases the CUD proved to be within or at the normal limits. As a control, we tested a patient with an agenetic posterior callosal defect due to a vascular malformation. In this case, the CUD was at the upper limits but still within the normal range, suggesting at least two possible alternatives: (a) neither the anterior, nor the posterior part of the corpus callosum are crucial for granting the interhemispheric integration of simple visuomotor responses; or (b) data from the last patient must be interpreted with caution, not only because they come from a single case, but also because the topographic organization of her partially agenetic corpus callosum may be abnormal: the fibres normally running in the splenium could have been re-addressed through more anterior portions of the corpus callosum (as shown experimentally in mice by Olavarria *et al.*, 1994). Yet there is evidence that callosal connections in the above case are functionally abnormal, since along with a normal CUD she exhibits clear signs of visual and tactile interhemispheric disconnection: left hemifield alexia, and left hand anomia (Aglioti *et al.*, 1998). Finally, it must be considered that both anterior callosotomy and splenial agenesis could spare connections between parietal areas, which in turn could be crucial for visuomotor integration (Anzola & Vignolo, 1992).

Attention and the split-brain

We have seen that the distinction between 'perceptual disunity and behavioural unity' (Sergent, 1987, p. 1375) needs some qualification. Let we consider now the statement by Gazzaniga (1987), that visual attention may be unified in the split-brain, even if visual perception is not. Of course, this would advance our understanding of the apparent unity of consciousness in the split-brain, since attention, no matter how defined, constitutes at least an important part of consciousness.

In vision, attention has often been likened to a 'spotlight' that enlightens selectively the portion of visual field where the processing of information is enhanced, without fixating eye movements, which would simply exploit the best sensory acuity. Experimentally, it is possible to measure how a subject can focus his attention by cueing him to expect a signal in a particular location. The response to a target will be speeded if it coincides with the cued location (benefits), and slowed if it does not (costs), relative to a neutral condition in which there is no cue. Holtzman *et al.* (1981) showed that in commissurotomy patients the decision whether a digit was even or odd was speeded when the place of its occurrence in a 3 x 3 grid was cued (either in the same or in the opposite hemifield), and slowed when the digit appeared in a non-cued location. This result is in agreement with the evidence by Holtzman himself (1984), that a callosotomized subject could direct an eye movement to a location in one hemifield on the basis of information presented in the other hemifield. Oculomotor responses and attentional preparation are closely linked, both being components of the orienting response to a lateralized stimulus. It should be noted also that in Holtzman *et al.* (1981), presenting in the two hemifields cues pointing in opposite directions had the same effect as presenting no cues (neutral situation), thus suggesting that the two hemispheres are not independent in accessing attentional resources, but must share a common substrate.

To complicate things, however, there is more recent evidence that, under given conditions, attention can be divided between the hemispheres. It is possible, and even easier, to orient attention by means of sensory rather than symbolic cues, consisting in the simple brightening of a box where successively the target is flashed with a high probability. With this paradigm, Reuter-Lorenz & Fendrich (1990) showed that callosotomized subjects benefited from ipsilateral but not contralateral cues, that is, each hemisphere proved to maintain a degree of attentional autonomy.

In a similar situation, Mangun *et al.* (1994) showed that split-brain patients benefited from a peripheral, sensory cue both for unilateral and bilateral brightenings, suggesting that attention can be divided in the two hemispheres, at variance with what happens to normals, and also to callosotomized patients with symbolic cues (see above). To further confirm that in this situation the two hemispheres behave independently, the performance appears to be different by considering separately the left hemifield, controlled by the right hemisphere, and the right hemifield,

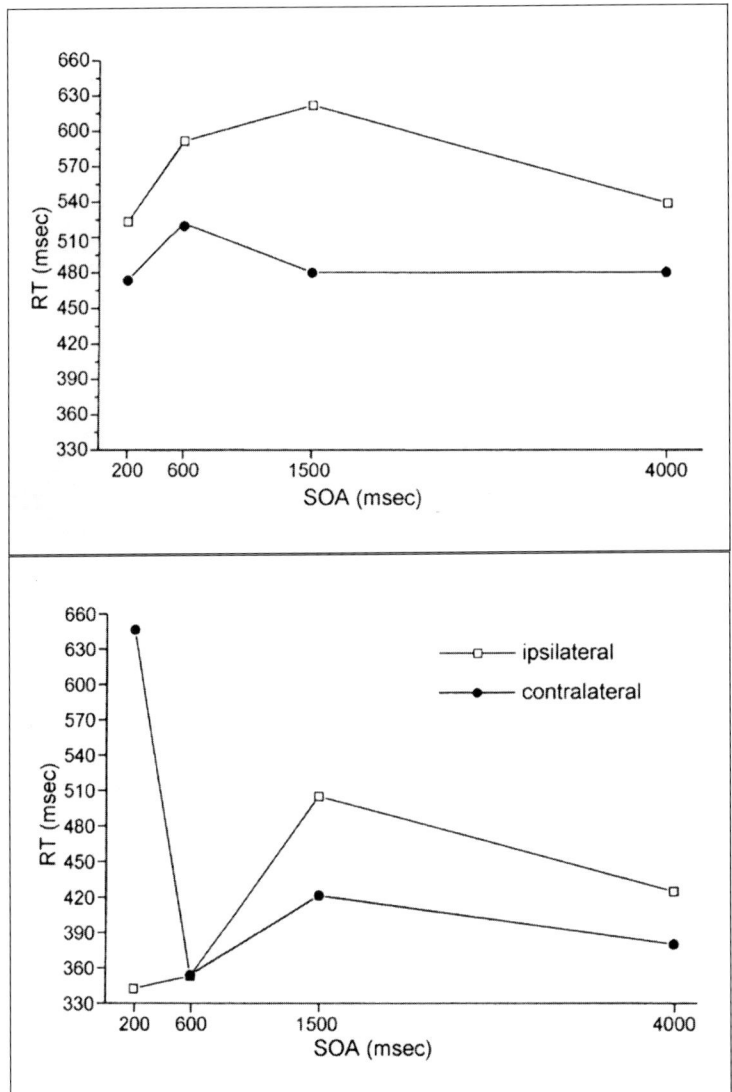

Fig. 4. Reaction time (RT) of a callosotomized subject as a function of the positional relationship between cue and target (ipsilateral, white squares, versus contralateral, black circles) and the stimulus onset asynchrony (SOA) between cue and target. Top and bottom panels correspond to location of the target in the left and right hemifield (modified from Berlucchi et al., 1997).

controlled by the left hemisphere. In the latter case, there are no costs, suggesting that the left hemisphere attended to the right hemifield regardless of cueing.

We have shown a similar, relative independence of the two hemispheres in the attentional processes of a callosotomized patient (Berlucchi et al., 1997). Not only did we use peripheral, sensory cues, but also a relation of non-predictivity between cues and targets: a flash of light in one of four locations could be followed by another flash of light in one of the same four locations, in the same hemifield or across midline. In normal subjects, this paradigm entails slowing of the responses when the two successive stimuli fall on the same point or anyhow on the same side of fixation as compared to when they fall on opposite sides. This is due to a process similar to the inhibition of return that has been described by Posner & Cohen (1984). The results of the callosotomized patient differ from that of normals for two important aspects. First, there is an effect of cue position, in addiction to the effect of target position, and for both cues and targets there is an advantage of the right over the left hemifield. Second, the attentional effect is asymmetric, as in Mangun et al. (1994): in the left hemifield the time course of ipsilateral inhibition and contralateral facilitation is similar to that of normal controls, while in the right hemifield there is an initial advantage, instead of a disadvantage, for ipsilateral cue-target combinations (Fig. 4).

It can be hypothesized that at the shortest cue-target interval the information of the right target, through the intrahemispheric pathway, reaches the decisional left hemisphere shortly after the information of the left cue (which has been delayed due to the slowed interhemispheric transfer), when the left hemisphere is fully refractory for the processing of another stimulus (psychological refractory period, Welford, 1980).

A combination of left hemisphere dominance and dissociation between implicit and explicit information processing can be seen if the callosotomized patient is simply requested to detect single and double, bilateral lights (Marzi *et al.*, 1997). The patient shows, through verbal response, extinction of the stimuli presented in the left hemifield along with those presented in the right hemifield; however, he is faster, like normal controls, in response to bilateral presentations, due to a summation effect.

Finally, a separated activity of the two hemispheres is confirmed by experiments that can be considered precursor of those concerning object-based, opposed to spatially selective, attention. Levy *et al.* (1972), using chimeric faces composed of two different halves, and suddenly reversing the response instruction, found that commissurotomized patients were able to attend simultaneously to the two half-faces.

Summing up, we started from a kind of functional amputation of some relations with half of the external world (left alexia, apraxia, anomia), and somehow paradoxically we conclude with functions which are left almost intact or downright duplicated by the division of the brain in its two halves.

References

Aglioti, S., Berlucchi, G., Pallini, R., Rossi, G.F. & Tassinari, G. (1993): Hemispheric control of unilateral and bilateral responses to lateralized light stimuli after callosotomy and in callosal agenesis. *Exp. Brain Res.* **95**, 151–165.

Aglioti, S., Beltramello, A., Tassinari, G. & Berlucchi, G. (1998): Paradoxically greater interhemispheric transfer deficits in partial than complete callosal agenesis. *Neuropsychologia* **36**, 1015–1024.

Akelaitis, A.J. (1944): A study of gnosis, praxis and language following section of the corpus callosum and anterior commissure. *J. Neurosurg.* **1**, 94–102.

Anzola, G.P. & Vignolo, L.A. (1992): Interhemispheric communication following unilateral cerebrovascular lesions. *Ital. J. Neurol. Sci.* **13**, 649–655.

Berlucchi, G., Crea, F., Di Stefano, M. & Tassinari, G. (1977): Influence of spatial stimulus-response compatibility on reaction time of ipsilateral and contralateral hand to lateralized light stimuli. *J. Exp. Psychol. Hum. Percept. Perform.* **3**, 505–517.

Berlucchi, G., Aglioti, S. & Tassinari, G. (1997): Rightward attentional bias and left hemisphere dominance in a cue-target light detection task in a callosotomy patient. *Neuropsychologia* **35**, 941–952.

Berlucchi, G.& Aglioti, S. (1999): Interhemispheric disconnection syndromes. In: *Handbook of neuropsychology*, eds. G. Denes & L. Pizzamiglio, pp. 635–670. Hove: Psychology Press.

Bogen, J.E. & Vogel, P.J. (1962): Cerebral commissurotomy in man. Preliminary case report. *Bull. Los Angeles Neurol. Soc.* **27**, 169.

Bykov, K.M. & Speranski, A.D. (1924): Observation upon dogs after section of the corpus callosum. In: *Collected papers physiology laboratories,* ed. I.P. Pavlov, vol. I, pp.47–59.

Carmant, L. & Holmes, G.L. (1994): Commissurotomies in children. *J. Child Neurol.* **9**, S2, 50–60.

Cendes, F., Ragazzo, P.C., da Costa, V. & Martins, L.F. (1993): Corpus callosotomy in treatment of medically resistant epilepsy: preliminary results in a pediatric population. *Epilepsia* **34**, 910–917.

Clarke, J.M. & Zaidel, E. (1989): Simple reaction times to lateralized light flashes: Varieties of interhemispheric communication routes. *Brain* **112,** 849–870.

Corballis, M.C. (1994): Can commissurotomy subjects compare digits between the visual fields? *Neuropsychologia* **32,** 1475–1486.

Corballis, M.C. (1995): Visual integration in the split-brain. *Neuropsychologia* **33,** 937–959.

Déjerine, J. (1892): Contribution à l'étude anatomo-pathologique et clinique des différentes variétés de cécité verbale. *Comptes Rendus de Séances et Mémoires de la Société de Biologie* **4,** 61–90.

Di Stefano, M., Morelli, M., Marzi, C.A. & Berlucchi, G. (1980): Hemispheric control of unilateral and bilateral movements of proximal and distal parts of the arms as inferred from simple reaction time to lateralized light stimuli in man. *Exp. Brain Res.* **38,** 197–204.

Fechner, G.T. (1889): *Elemente der Psychophysik*, vol. II, Leipzig: Breitkopf und Härtel.

Fiol, M.E., Gates, J.R., Mireles, R., Maxwell, R.E. & Erickson, D.M. (1993): Value of intraoperative EEG changes during corpus callosotomy in predicting surgical results. *Epilepsia* **34,** 74–78.

Freund, C.S. (1889): Ueber optische Aphasie und Seelenblindheit. *Archiv fur Psychiatrie und Nervenkrankheiten* **20,** 276–297, 371–416.

Fuiks, K.S., Wyler, A.R., Hermann, B.P. & Somes, G. (1991): Seizure outcome from anterior and complete corpus callosotomy. *J. Neurosurg.* **74,** 573–578.

Gazzaniga, M.S., Bogen, J.E. & Sperry, R.W. (1962): Some functional effects of sectioning the cerebral commissures in man. *Proc. Nat. Acad. Sci. USA* **48,** 1765–1769.

Gazzaniga, M.S. (1987): Perceptual and attentional processes following callosal section in humans. *Neuropsychologia* **25,** 119–133.

Gazzaniga, M.S. & Smylie, C.S. (1990): Hemispheric mechanisms controlling voluntary and spontaneous facial expressions. *J. Cogn. Neurosci.* **2,** 239–245.

Gozzano, M. (1935): Ricerche sui fenomeni elettrici della corteccia cerebrale. *Rivista di Neurologia* **8,** 212–261.

von Hartman, E. (1871): *Philosophie des Unbewussten*. Berlin: Carl Dunckers.

Holtzman, J.D., Sidtis, J.J., Volpe, B.T., Wilson, D.H. & Gazzaniga, M.S. (1981): Dissociation of spatial information for stimulus localization and control of attention. *Brain* **104,** 861–872.

Holtzman, J.D. (1984): Interactions between cortical and subcortical visual areas: evidence from human commissurotomy patients. *Vis. Res.* **8,** 801–813.

Jeeves, M.A. (1990): Agenesis of the corpus callosum. In: *Handbook of neuropsychology*, eds. F. Boller & J. Grafman, vol. 4, pp. 99–114. Amsterdam: Elsevier.

Kuypers, H.G.J.M. (1981): Anatomy of the descending pathways. In: *Handbook of physiology,* Section I: The nervous system, eds. J.M. Brookhart & V.B. Mountcastle, vol. II: *Motor Control*, ed. V.B. Brooks, pp. 597–666. Bethesda MD: American Physiology Society.

Lashley, K.S. (1951): The problem of serial order in behavior. In: *Cerebral mechanisms in behavior: the Hixon symposium*, ed. L.P. Jeffress, pp. 112–136. New York: Wiley.

Lassonde, M., Sauerwein, H., Geoffroy, G. & Décarie, M. (1986): Effects of early and late transection of the corpus callosum in children. A study of tactile and tactuomotor transfer and integration. *Brain* **109,** 953–967.

Lassonde, M., Sauerwein, H., McCabe, N., Laurencelle, L. & Geoffroy, G. (1988): Extent and limits of cerebral adjustment to early section or congenital absence of the corpus callosum. *Behav. Brain Res.* **30,** 165–181.

Lassonde, M., Sauerwein, H., Chicoine, A.J. & Geoffroy, G. (1991): Absence of disconnexion syndrome in callosal agenesis and early callosotomy: brain reorganization or lack of structural specificity during ontogeny? *Neuropsychologia* **29,** 481–495.

Lassonde, M. & Sauerwein, H. (1997): Neuropsychological outcome of corpus callosotomy in children and adolescents. *J. Neurosurg. Sci.* **41,** 67–73.

Levy, J., Trevarthen, C. & Sperry, R.W. (1972): Perception of bilateral chimeric figures following hemispheric deconnection. *Brain* **95,** 61–78.

Liepmann, H. (1900): Das Krankheitsbild der Apraxie ('Motorischen Asymbolie') auf Grund eines Falles von einseitiger Apraxie. *Monatschrift für Psychiatrie und Neurologie* **8**, 15–44, 102–132, 182–197.

Mamelak, A.N., Barbaro, N.M., Walker, J.A. & Laxer, K.D. (1993): Corpus callosotomy: a quantitative study of the extent of resection, seizure control, and neuropsychological outcome. *J. Neurosurg.* **79**, 688–695.

Mangun, G.R., Luck, S.J., Plager, R., Loftus, W., Hillyard, S.A., Handy, T., Clark, V.P. & Gazzaniga, M.S. (1994): Monitoring the visual world: hemispheric asymmetries and subcortical processes in attention. *J. Cogn. Neurosci.* **6**, 267–275.

Marzi, C.A., Fanini, A., Girelli, M., Ipata, A.E., Miniussi, C., Prior, M. & Smania, N. (1997): Is extinction following parietal damage an interhemispheric disconnection phenomenon? In: *Parietal lobe contribution to orientation in 3D space*, eds. P. Their & H.O. Karnath, pp. 431–445. Heidelberg: Springer.

McCulloch, W. (1949): Mechanisms for the spread of epileptic activation of the brain. *Electroencephal. Clin. Neurophysiol.* **1**, 19–24.

Milner, A.D., Jeeves, M.A., Silver, P.H., Lines, C.R. & Wilson, J. (1985): Reaction times to lateralized visual stimuli in callosal agenesis: stimulus and response factors. *Neuropsychologia* **23**, 323–331.

Moruzzi, G. (1939): Contribution à l'électrophysiologie du cortex moteur. Facilitation, after-discharge et épilepsie corticale. *Arch. Internat. Physiol.* **49**, 33–100.

Myers, R.E. & Sperry, R.W. (1953): Interocular transfer of a visual form discrimination habit in cats after section of the optic chiasma and corpus callosum. *Anat. Rec.* **115**, 351–352.

Nordgren, R.E., Reeves, A.G., Viguera, A.C. & Roberts, D.W. (1991): Corpus callosotomy for intractable seizures in the pediatric age group. *Arch. Neurol.* **48**, 364–372.

Oguni, H., Olivier, A., Andermann, F. & Comair, J. (1991): Anterior callosotomy in the treatment of medically intractable epilepsies: a study of 43 patients with a mean follow-up of 39 months. *Ann. Neurol.* **30**, 357–364.

Olavarria, J., Serra-Oller, M.M., Yee, K.T. & Van Sluyters, R.C. (1994): Pattern of interhemispheric connections in mice with congenital deficiencies of the corpus callosum. In: *Callosal agenesis: a natural split-brain?*, eds. M. Lassonde & M.A. Jeeves, pp. 135–146. New York: Plenum Press.

Pallini, R., Aglioti, S., Tassinari, G., Berlucchi, G., Colosimo, C. & Rossi, G.F. (1995): Corpus callosotomy for intractable epilepsy from bihemispheric cortical dysplasias. *Acta Neurochirugica* **132**, 79–86.

Papo, I., Quattrini, A., Ortenzi, A., Paggi, A., Rychlicki, F., Provinciali, L. Del Pesce, M., Cesarano, C. & Fioravanti, P. (1997): Predictive factors of callosotomy in drug-resistant epileptic patients with a long follow-up. *J. Neurosurg. Sci.* **41**, 31–36.

Poffenberger, A.T. (1912): Reaction time to retinal stimulation with special reference to the time lost in conduction through nervous centers. *Arch. Psychol.* **23**, 1–73.

Posner, M.I & Cohen, Y. (1984): Components of visual orienting. In: *Attention and performance*, eds. H. Bouma & G.G. Bouwhuis, pp. 531–556. Hillsdale, NJ: Erlbaum.

Ramachandran, V.S., Cronin-Golomb, A & Myers, J.J. (1986): Perception of apparent motion by commissurotomy patients. *Nature* **320**, 358–359.

Reutens, D.C., Bye, A.M., Hopkins, I.J., Danks, A., Somerville, E., Walsh, J., Bleasel, A., Ouvrier, R., MacKenzie, R.A., Manson, J.I., Bladin, P.F. & Berkovic, S.F. (1993): Corpus callosotomy for intractable epilepsy: seizure outcome and prognostic factors. *Epilepsia* **34**, 904–909.

Reuter-Lorenz, P.A. & Fendrich, R. (1990): Orienting attention across the vertical meridian: evidence from callosotomy patients. *J. Cogn. Neurosci.* **2**, 232–238.

Ringo, J.L., Doty, R.W., Demeter, S. & Simard, P.Y. (1994): Time is of the essence: a conjecture that hemispheric specialization arises from interhemispheric conduction delay. *Cer. Cortex* **4**, 331–343.

Rugg, M.D., Lines, C.R. & Milner, A.D. (1984): Visual evoked potentials to lateralized visual stimuli and the measurement of interhemispheric transmission time. *Neuropsychologia* **22**, 215–225.

Sergent, J. (1983): Unified response to bilateral hemispheric stimulation by a split-brain patient. *Nature* **305**, 800–802.

Sergent, J. (1986): Subcortical coordination of hemisphere activity in commissurotomized patients. *Brain* **109**, 357–369.

Sergent, J. (1987): A new look at the human split brain. *Brain* **110**, 1375–1392.

Sergent, J. & Myers, J.J. (1985): Manual, blowing, and verbal simple reactions to lateralized flashes of light in commissurotomized patients. *Percept. Psychophys.* **37**, 571–578.

Spencer, S.S., Spencer, D.D., Sass, K, Westerveld, M., Katz, A. & Mattson, R. (1993): Anterior, total and two-stage corpus callosum section: differential and incremental seizure responses. *Epilepsia* **34**, 561–567.

Sperry, R.W., Gazzaniga, M.S. & Bogen, J.E. (1969): Interhemispheric relationships: the neocortical commissures; syndromes of hemispheric disconnection. In: *Handbook of clinical neurology*, vol. 4, *Disorders of speech, perception, and symbolic behaviour*, eds. P.J. Vinken & G.W. Bruyn, pp. 273–290. Amsterdam: Elsevier.

Sugishita, M., Shinohara, A., Shimoji, T. & Ogawa, T. (1985): A remaining problem in hemialexia: tachistoscopic hemineglect and hemialexia. In: *Epilepsy and the corpus callosum*, ed. A.G. Reeves, pp. 417–434. New York: Plenum Press.

Tassinari, G., Aglioti, S., Pallini, R., Berlucchi, G. & Rossi, G.F. (1994): Interhemispheric integration of visuomotor responses in patients with partial callosal defects. *Behav. Brain Res.* **64**, 141–149.

Trevarthen, C. & Sperry, R.W. (1973): Perceptual unity of the ambient visual field in human commissurotomy patients. *Brain* **96**, 547–570.

Van Wagenen, W.P. & Herren, R.Y. (1940): Surgical division of commissural pathways in the corpus callosum. *Arch. Neurol. Psychiat.* **44**, 740–759.

Welford, A.T. (1980): The single-channel hypothesis. In: *Reaction times*, ed. A.T. Welford, pp. 215–252. London: Academic Press.

Wilson, D.H., Culver, C., Waddington, M. & Gazzaniga, M.S. (1975): Disconnection of the cerebral hemispheres. An alternative to hemispherectomy for the control of intractable seizures. *Neurology* **25**, 1149–1153.

Chapter 6

Basal ganglia lesions, language and neuropsychological dysfunction

Isabel Pavão Martins

Department of Neurology, Centro de Estudos Egas Moniz, Hospital de Sta Maria, 1600 Lisbon, Portugal

Summary

There is not much knowledge about the behavioural consequences of subcortical and basal ganglia lesions during childhood. In this paper we review the literature on this subject, and present a series of cases illustrating different neuropsychological syndromes associated with subcortical damage in children under 15 years of age. There is a trend for 'anterior' left hemisphere lesions to be associated with more severe language difficulties than posterior lesions. However, even in small series of patients, there are atypical anatomo-clinical associations and the observed behaviour depends not only on lesion localization and size, but also on the indirect and transient effects of such lesions upon the overlying cortex. There were no cases of severe and longstanding behavioural and emotional disturbances suggesting a minor contribution of subcortical structures to emotional behaviour in children. While the acute syndromes were identical to the ones described in adult patients, recovery in children was quite fast, suggesting that the undamaged cortical areas may easily compensate for their dysfunction.

Introduction

Located deep in the cerebral hemispheres there is a group of grey matter nuclei called the basal ganglia. These include, among others, the *caudate nucleus*, the *lenticular nucleus* (with an outer part called the *putamen* and an inner part, the *globus pallidus*) and a larger and more posterior nucleus, the *thalamus*. While the first two are involved in motor functions, they are part of the extrapyramidal system, the latter receives all the sensory information travelling into the brain.

In between these nuclei there are multiple white matter fibre tracts, carrying fibres travelling in and out of the cerebral cortex to the brainstem, basal ganglia and the spinal cord. Among these tracts there is the *internal capsule* (IC) (with an anterior and a posterior limb and a middle part, the genu), the *temporal isthmus* (TI) (carrying fibres from the medial geniculate body to the auditory cortex), the *periventricular white matter* (PVWM) located around the lateral ventricles, and the *medial subcallosal fasciculus* (ScF) (with fibres from the cingular gyrus and the supplementary motor area, located in the inner part of the frontal lobe, to the head of the caudate nucleus).

These subcortical structures are connected to each other and to the cerebral cortex in multiple and complex ways but, in general, the fibres travel from the different parts of the cortex to the striatum (name given both to the caudate and the putamen), from there they project into the pallidus, from the pallidus they travel to the thalamus and from there they go back to the cortex. These loops are called the cortico-striato-pallido-thalamo-cortical loops, which subserve multiple functions. Some of them have an activating or modulatory role on the overlying cortex.

These structures are concentrated in a relatively small area of the brain. Therefore any small lesion can damage more than one of them. This is particularly important in vascular lesions, because each one of the vascular territories supplies more than one of those anatomical structures. This makes it difficult to study the individual role of each of these structures in specific functions or symptoms.

For many years the basal ganglia were though to be responsible for motor functions only. However, with the advent of brain imaging (CT and MRI scans) it became clear that deep hemisphere lesions could interfere with behaviour. The first studies on this matter were published in the early 1980s on adult patients with deep hemispheric stroke and focused on language and hemispatial neglect (Watson *et al.*, 1981; Damásio *et al.*, 1982; Naeser *et al.*, 1982). But soon other papers followed, describing cases of memory, behavioural and emotional disturbances (Habib & Poncet, 1988; Mendez *et al.*, 1989). Animal experiments corroborated the role of these structures in a variety of cognitive functions and behaviour (Divac & Oberg, 1992).

Attempts were made to correlate each anatomical area to a function or syndrome. However, this was controversial. Some authors (Basso *et al.*, 1987) could not find such a correlation, while others (Naeser *et al.*, 1982; Alexander *et al.*, 1987; Naeser *et al.*, 1989; Mega & Alexander, 1994) have drawn models of the relations between some of these areas and specific linguistic defects or behavioural dysfunction.

The difficulty in establishing such clinico-anatomical correlations is not just due to the fact that single lesions (particularly the vascular ones) tend to damage multiple areas. The main methodological problem is that the symptoms caused by purely subcortical lesions can result from different pathogenic mechanisms. The basal ganglia have a direct effect on behaviour since they integrate cortico-subcortical neuronal networks subserving language and other complex behaviours. But these structures may also have an indirect effect upon cognitive functions, as they may produce a depression of the metabolic activity of the overlying cortex, as has been demonstrated with the PET scan (Metter *et al.*, 1988).

In contrast with the extensive research on subcortical damage in adults, there is not much knowledge on the role of the basal ganglia in childhood.

One of the reasons for that is probably because stroke, which is the main cause of subcortical damage in adults, is rare during childhood. But there are other reasons.

1. Firstly, clinical reports do not always mention neuropsychological assessment. For instance in a review of 104 cases of subcortical stroke in childhood that were published in the English literature in the last 20 years (Powell *et al.*, 1994), there is no mention of language or cognitive dysfunction. In two other studies (Zimmerman *et al.*, 1983; Sahar *et al.*, 1990),

totalling 30 cases, there are eight patients with 'language or mental status change' especially in association with large infarcts. Language disorder is not described.

2. Secondly, published series of children with aphasia or other cognitive disorders often do not describe lesion localization in detail. In particular, a differentiation is not always made between cortical and subcortical damage.

3. Thirdly, even in series of childhood aphasia where lesion localization is described, there are very few analyses (Aram & Ekelman, 1988) of the independent effect of a subcortical localization.

To these difficulties, we must add the usual constraints one finds when studying behavioural disorders in children: in a small series of patients one has to consider a large number of variables, some of which related to the subject (handedness, educational level, socio-economic status, familiar status), other variables are related to the lesion (aetiology, localization and size, associated disorders) and still others to 'timing' (the age at lesion onset, but also the time post onset) since there is always some change with time which, in children, can be dramatic in a few days. Besides, there are differences in methodology depending upon the child's age and the authors perspective (clinical, cognitive or neurolinguistic approach).

Therefore one often has to rely upon the analysis of individual cases rather than studying the effects of specific sites of lesion (as has been done in adult patients).

I shall try to review here the extant data on this subject, looking separately at the effect of left and right subcortical lesions.

Subcortical lesions of the left hemisphere

There are at least some 18 published cases of subcortical aphasia in children (Table 1).

Table 1. Subcortical aphasia in acquired aphasia series

Author, year	Total number of cases	Subcortical cases	Subcortical aphasia
Van Hout *et al.*, 1985	11	nil	nil
Vargha Khadem *et al.*, 1985	20	?	not recorded
Cramberg *et al.*, 1987	8	1	1
Van Dongen *et al.*, 1990	30	2	2
Toshiko *et al.*, 1990	3	nil	nil
Lees and Neville, 1990	5	nil	nil
Aram, 1992	> 30	9	7
Martins, 1993	99	14	6

These cases were described either in series of patients with acquired aphasia (Cramberg *et al.*, 1987; Loonen & Van Dongen, 1990; Martins & Ferro, 1993) or as case reports (Ferro *et al.*, 1982; Aram *et al.*, 1983; Picard *et al.*, 1989; Markowitsch *et al.*, 1990; Aram & Eisele, 1993; Martins & Ferro, 1992; Martins *et al.*, 1993).

It is altogether a small number of patients, and we do not know if the percentage of aphasia following subcortical damage in children is more or less frequent than in adults. The exact prevalence could only be recognized if we had data on the negative cases as well, but there are many more reports on positive than on negative cases.

Reviewing those cases we can see that the presentation is not homogeneous and multiple syndromes may result. There is usually a period of mutism followed by motor disorders of speech (dysarthria, dysprosodia and hypophonia) and an aphasia, fluent or nonfluent, with normal or impaired verbal comprehension. Word finding difficulties are usual, and literal and semantic paraphasias have been reported.

Aram & Eiselle (1993) divided their patients by an anterior/posterior anatomical axis. According to these authors, 'anterior' lesions tend to produce nonfluent types of speech and good auditory comprehension. 'Posterior lesions', on the other hand, may cause comprehension disorders, fluent aphasia (conduction type) or no aphasia at all. In both locations there are motor disorders of speech (dysarthria and hypophonia), and both have a good prognosis for total recovery. On the contrary, if the lesion involves simultaneously the anterior and the posterior subcortical structures, then the defects are more severe and persistent. Several years after the lesion, these patients remain dysfluent and obtain low scores in several language measures.

This division is identical to the one described in adult patients (Naeser et al., 1982; Mega & Alexander 1994). According to these authors the symptoms depend on the damaged loops. 'Anterior' lesions tend to interrupt three main anatomical loops:

(a) motor loops (including the putamen, middle PVWM or the genu of the IC), producing motor speech defects,

(b) loops involved in motor initiation (with fibres travelling from the prefrontal cortex, anterior cingulate gyrus and suplementary motor area to the caudate nucleus through the ScF) which damage causes mutism, hypokinesia and hypophonia, and

(c) loops responsible for lexical access and generative aspects of language, whose damage produces aphasia and word finding difficulties.

On the other hand, 'posterior' lesions tend to interrupt the auditory pathways in the temporal isthmus, or their projections to the caudate nucleus causing disorders of verbal auditory comprehension and Wernicke's type of aphasia (Damasio et al., 1982).

In a total of 13 patients with purely subcortical lesions sustained before the 15th birthday, personally observed by the author, there were five patients with aphasia (Table 2).

Most of them have 'anterior' lesions. While the majority of them are in accordance with the proposed model of anatomoclinical correlation, others are quite atypical.

Table 2. Subcortical aphasia

No.	Age	Sex	Aetiology	Mutism	Aphasia Type	Caudate nucleus	Putamen	Anterior IC	Posterior IC	Corona radiata
1	2.7	F	ischaemic	+	Broca					+
2	15	F	haematoma	+	Transcortical Motor	+	+	+		
3	9.3	M	trauma	+	Transcortical Motor		+	+		
4	11	F	haematoma	−	Anomic		+	+		
5	13	M	ischaemic	−	Anomic	+		+		

F = female; M = male; IC = internal capsula.

The first patient (Patient 1, Table 2) (Martins & Ferro, 1992) is a 2-year-old girl who had an infarct involving the PVWM, specially its anterior and superior parts, visible on a single cut on CT scan. This child had a transient nonfluent aphasia, lasting 3 days and a total recovery. Her last neuropsychological assessment, performed when she was 9 years old, was entirely normal, and she was doing very well at school.

A second case (Patient 2), a 15-year-old-girl (Martins & Ferro, 1992), had a coagulation disorder, suffered an haematoma in the anterior putamen, anterior IC and caudate nucleus. She was mute for almost one month. This was followed by a nonfluent transcortical motor aphasia with good auditory comprehension and repetition, and a severe motor speech disorder with dysarthria, slow effortful speech and a flattened prosody. Eight months later she was no longer aphasic, but the speech disorder lasted at least 2.5 years and she went on to have writing difficulties at school.

Another case (Patient 3), a 9-year-old boy, suffered a left subcortical haemorrhage following a head trauma. He was in mutism for 40 days. Two months later he had a nonfluent speech that was slow monocordic, with a flattened prosody, and consisting of isolated words or short sentences with multiple pauses and occasional literal and semantic paraphasias. Comprehension and repetition were normal. He was classified as a transcortical motor aphasia. He recovered from this language disorder in 5 months but his speech remained slow and his writing was poor, specially to dictation.

So these three cases are typical cases of 'anterior' lesions: they have nonfluent aphasia, motor speech defects, and a good immediate outcome for aphasia recovery, although speech disturbances tend to last more than aphasia.

But the presentation can also be atypical. Two of our patients with 'anterior' lesions (cases 4 and 5) had fluent, anomic types of aphasia. Case 4, an 11-year-old girl had a spontaneous haematoma involving the head of the anterior putamen and the anterior limb of the IC. Her speech was fluent, though slightly dysarthric, from the onset of lesion. She had word-finding difficulties and semantic paraphasias. Object naming was poor but otherwise her language was normal. On the 7th day she was fully recovered from aphasia but her spontaneous writing was agrammatic. Two years later she was still having some writing difficulties and she developed a provocative and negative behaviour at school that was interfering with learning. But this was coincident with family problems, another variable to take into account when interpreting behavioural problems in children.

Case 5, a 13-year-old boy with an 'anterior' subcortical infarct, involving the head of the caudate nucleus (Martins et al., 1993) also had an anomic aphasia with a fluent speech with circumlocutions and clichés, atypical for such an 'anterior' lesion.

We have also seen patients with a 'posterior' subcortical involvement. All of them were negative cases for they were never aphasic (cases 6, 7 and 8).

Case 6, a 10-year-old-boy (Martins & Ferro, 1992) had an haematoma of the posterior limb of the IC due to a small arteriovenous malformation. He had no aphasia at all (he was fully assessed on the 5th day post onset).

Case 7, a 8-year-old girl suffered a posterior subcortical infarction following the endovascular occlusion of a middle cerebral artery aneurysm. She had a transient aphasia during the first attempt to inflate the intra-arterial balloon, thus demonstrating that language was lateralized to the left hemisphere in her case. That transient episode resolved completely when the balloon was deflated. However, hours later she developed a right sided hemiparesis and the CT scan showed an infarction involving the posterior putamen. This lesion did not cause any language disorder. Three years later, this girl is doing very well, having a normal performance at school.

Another patient, case 8, had a posterior subcortical bleeding from a deeply located arteriovenous malformation. There is no mention of any language disorder in the acute period. We examined this girl some 10 years later and she had no neuropsychological defects in tests of oral or written language or calculation abilities.

Two of the 'posterior' cases of Aram & Eisele (1993) also had normal neuropsychological evaluations. This results suggest that there may be more negative cases in the 'posterior' subcortical group, than in cases of 'anterior' damage. It is not clear why this happens.

One of our patients, case 5 (Martins et al., 1993) was investigated by a SPECT scan. This case helps us understand the pathogenesis and the variability of these syndromes. This boy had an 'anterior' subcortical infarct, involving the anterior limb of the internal capsule ant the head of the caudate nucleus. He had an anomic aphasia. Although he could follow simple verbal commands he had a very low score in the Token test (De Renzi & Vignolo, 1962) showing a disorder of auditory comprehension. His first cerebral SPECT scan was performed on the 9th day post onset, the same day of the first neuropsychological assessment. Although his lesion was small and deeply located in the left cerebral hemisphere, there was a profound decrease of the metabolic activity of the overlying cortex, especially over the frontal and temporal lobes. Three months later he was reassessed. His language performance was by then normal and another SPECT just showed a small dysfunctional area corresponding to the subcortical infarct. This case shows that at least some of the symptoms observed in association with subcortical lesions can be explained by a transient diaschisis, i.e. a distant and reversible defect between functionally connected, but intact, brain areas. We do not know what the importance of this phenomenon may be, and we need negative cases to understand it better. This boy was re-evaluated 3 years later. He was having problems at school, repeating one grade for the fourth time. The only neuropsychological sequelae found was a mild impairment of the short term verbal memory.

In conclusion, there is a great variability of clinical presentation of subcortical aphasia in children. This can result from small differences in lesion site or size. Size seems important, for lacunar infarctions in adults do not cause language dysfunction and aphasia has been reported to occur specially with large infarcts in children. Lesion site is also relevant, since small variations in lesions localization will interrupt different neuronal networks. Besides, variability can also result from the distant and transient effects of such lesions upon the cortex. In a study in adult patients with the PET Scan (Metter et al., 1988) it was found that the effect of subcortical lesions on comprehension is purely an indirect one, while the effect on fluency is both direct and indirect. Despite this variability, there is a trend for more anterior lesions to cause mutism and nonfluent transcortical motor or Broca type of aphasia with marked motor speech defects which may persist. 'Posterior' lesions tend to have no effects on language or to cause disorders of auditory comprehension or short term memory or dysarthria.

This general pattern is identical to what was described in adults, but there are some differences.

Firstly, 'posterior' lesions seem to cause aphasia less frequently and there are, so far, no reports of Wernicke type of aphasia in childhood due to subcortical damage. This suggests that auditory comprehension may be more dependent upon cortical than subcortical structures in this age group.

Secondly, there are no cases of profound behavioural disorders, as have been described in adults with caudate infarctions (abulia, indifference, depression, lack of initiative or frontal-lobe-like behaviour). We may speculate that this results from the immature development of the prefrontal connections in this age group.

The last difference concerns the prognosis, which is better in children. Indeed, the immediate recovery was quite good in most of the reported cases. It took place in days or months. This can be due, in part, to a reversible diaschisis, but the intact cortex is also important. We compared a group of children with purely subcortical aphasia to a control group of aphasics matched for age, aetiology and subcortical lesion site, but who had in addition a cortical involvement (Martins & Ferro, 1992). We found that the latter group had a more prolonged and severe aphasia, suggesting that language recovery depends more on the intact areas of the overlying cortex than upon language transfer to the right hemisphere. But this is the immediate outcome. If we look at the long term prognosis we have a different picture. In one study (Aram & Ekelman, 1988) it was found that these children, compared to controls, had a lower verbal IQ. In our cases, many went on to develop scholastic difficulties and writing disorders. Agraphia is an important sequelae of subcortical aphasia in adults as well (Kertesz, 1992) perhaps because these structures integrate semantic and graphemic information with motor control. Besides, the caudate nucleus is known to be involved in several tasks important for learning, such as habit forming, integration of memories, attention span and interest and motivation. Impairment of these functions may underlie these learning difficulties.

Subcortical lesions and the right hemisphere

The data concerning subcortical lesions of the right hemisphere in children are even more sparse than for left hemisphere lesions, so I will just discuss it in relation to some cases we have examined.

Case 9 is an 8-year-old-girl (Ferro & Martins, 1990) with a coagulation disorder (aplastic anaemia) who developed a right thalamic haematoma. On the acute stage she was drowsy and had a mild left hemiparesis but she recovered from this motor defect and was examined 1 month later. At that time it was noticed she tended not to use her left upper limb unless she was specifically requested. During simultaneous movements of both hands, she tended to forget the left hand movements, a phenomenon called 'motor' neglect. She also had a marked visuospatial impairment, but no visuospatial neglect.

Another patient, case 10, a 6-year-old left handed girl (Ferro *et al.*, 1982), suffered a right hemisphere infarction involving the posterior limb IC, the lenticular nucleus and the corona radiata. She had a nonfluent aphasia but she also had a visuospatial dysfunction: a left hemispatial neglect and a spatial dysgraphia. She recovered in 15 days.

The last patients are 'negative' cases. An 8-year-old girl (case 11) and a 11-year-old girl (case 12) had, both, right hemisphere subcortical haematomas following head trauma. There is no description of neglect in the acute stage in either of them. They were assessed, respectively, 3 years and 5 months post onset. Both had normal visuospatial abilities and no visual, tactile, motor or hemispatial neglect.

In conclusion: motor and visual neglect and visuospatial disturbances can occur in children following subcortical damage to the right hemisphere, just as in adults (Ferro *et al.*, 1987). However, children tend to recover quickly. If they are not examined in the acute stage of illness it is unlikely that these defects will be found. There seem to be no major long term effects, although Aram & Ekelman (1988) reported that these patients tend to have a performance IQ below verbal IQ, when compared to controls.

Conclusions

Subcortical structures are specialized from an early age: there are right/left differences, identical to the ones found in adults. One of the main differences of subcortical damage between adults and children is the better outcome for immediate recovery in the latter. However, long term effects can occur, specially when children were aphasic in the acute stage (in particular, learning difficulties). The pathogenesis of symptoms observed in association with subcortical damage probably involves direct mechanisms and indirect effects upon the overlying cortex.

References

Alexander, M.P., Naeser, M.A. & Palumbo, C.L. (1987): Correlations of subcortical CT lesion sites and aphasia profiles. *Brain* **110,** 961–991.

Aram, D.M., Rose, D.F., Rekate, H.L. & Whitaker, H.A. (1983): Acquired capsular/striatal aphasia in childhood. *Arch. Neurol.* **40,** 614–617.

Aram, D.M. & Ekelman, B.L. (1988): Scholastic aptitude and achievement among children with unilateral brain lesions. *Neuropsychologia* **26,** 903–916.

Aram, D. & Eisele, J. (1993): Language development following subcortical lesions in children. Paper presented at the European Meeting of the International Neuropsychological Society, Funchal, Portugal.

Basso, A., Della Sala, S. & Farabola, M. (1987): Aphasia arising from purely deep lesions. *Cortex* **23,** 29–44.

Cramberg, L.D., Filley, C.M., Hart, E.J. & Alexander, M.P. (1987): Acquired aphasia in childhood: clinical and CT investigations. *Neurology* **37,** 1165–1172.

Damásio, A.R., Damásio, H., Rizzo, M., Varney, N. & Gersh, F. (1982). Aphasia with nonhemorrhagic lesions in the basal ganglia and internal capsule. *Arch. Neurol.* **39,** 15–20.

De Renzi, E. & Vignolo, L.A. (1962): The token test: a sensitive test to detect receptive disturbances in aphasics. *Brain* **85,** 665–678.

Divac, I. & Oberg, R.G.E. (1992): Subcortical mechanisms in cognition. In: *Neuropsychological disorders associated with subcortical lesions,* eds. G. Vallar, S.F. Cappa & Claus-W. Wallesch, pp. 42–60. Oxford: Oxford University Press.

Ferro, J.M., Martins, I.P., Castro-Caldas, A. & Pinto, F. (1982): Aphasia following right striato-insular infarction in a left handed child. A clinico-radiological study. *Develop. Med. Child Neurol.* **24,** 173–182.

Ferro, J.M., Kertesz, A. & Black, S.E. (1987): Subcortical neglect: quantitation, anatomy and recovery. *Neurology* **37,** 1487–1492.

Ferro, J.M. & Martins, I.P. (1990): Some new aspects of neglect in children. *Behav. Neurol.* **3,** 1–6.

Habib, M. & Poncet, M. (1988). Perte de l'élan vital, de l'intérêt et de l'affectivité (syndrome athymhormique) au cours de lésions lacunaires des des corps striés. *Rev. Neurol.* **144,** 5 71–577.

Kertesz, A. (1992). Subcortical agraphia. In: *Neuropsychological disorders associated with subcortical lesions,* eds. G. Vallar, S.F. Cappa & Claus-W. Wallesch, pp. 344–356. Oxford: Oxford University Press.

Loonen, M.C.B. & Van Dongen, H. (1990): Acquired childhood aphasia. Outcome one year after onset. *Arch. Neurol.* **47,** 1324–1328.

Markowitsch, H.J., Von Cramon, D.Y., Hofmann, E., Sick, C.D. & Kinzler, P. (1990). Verbal memory deterioration after unilateral infarct of the internal capsule in an adolescent. *Cortex* **26,** 597–609.

Martins, I.P. (1993): *Cortical brain damage in childhood.* Paper presented at the European Meeting of the International Neuropsychological Society, Funchal, Portugal.

Martins, I.P. & Ferro, J.M. (1992): Acquired subcortical lesions in children. In: *Neuropsychological disorders associated with subcortical lesions*, eds. G. Vallar, S.F. Cappa & Claus-W. Wallesch, pp. 381–396. Oxford: Oxford University Press, Oxford.

Martins, I.P., Ferro, J.M. & Cantinho, G. (1993): Acquired childhood aphasia, temporal lobe dysfunction and comprehension disorders. Paper presented at the European Meeting of the International Neuropsychological Society, Funchal, Portugal.

Martins, I.P. & Ferro, J.M. (1993): Acquired childhood aphasia: a clinicoradiological study of 11 stroke patients. *Aphasiology* **7**, 489–495.

Mega, M.S. & Alexander, M.P. (1994): Subcortical aphasia: the core profile of capsulostriatal infarction. *Neurology* **44**, 1824–1829.

Mendez, M.F., Adams, N.I. & Lewandowski, K.S. (1989). Neurobehavioural changes associated with caudate lesions. *Neurology* **39**, 349–354.

Metter, E.J., Riege, W.H., Hanson, W.R., Jackson, C.A., Kempler, D. & Lancker, D. (1988): Subcortical structures in aphasia. An analysis based on (F-18) fluorodeoxyglucose, positron emission tomography and computed tomography. *Arch. Neurol.* **45**, 1229–1234.

Naeser, M.A., Alexander, M.P., Helm-Estabrooks, N., Levine, H., Laughlin, S.A. & Geschwind, N. (1982): Aphasia with predominantly subcortical lesions sites. Description of three capsular/putaminal aphasia syndromes. *Arch. Neurol.* **39**, 2–14.

Naeser, M.A., Palumbo, C.L., Helm-Estabrooks, N., Stiassny-Eder, D. & Albert, M.L. (1989): Severe non-fluency in aphasia. *Brain* 112, 1–38.

Picard, A., Elghozi, D., Schouman-Claeys, E. & Lacert, P.H. (1989): Troubles du langage de type sous-cortical et hémidystonie séquelles d'un infarctus putamino-caudé datant de la première enfance. *Rev. Neurol.* **145**, 73–75.

Powell, F.C., Hanigan, C. & McCluney, K.W. (1994): Subcortical infarction in children. *Stroke* **25**, 117–121.

Sahar, E., Gilday, D.L., Hwang, P.A., Cohen, E.K. & Lambert, R. (1990): Pediatric cerebrovascular disease. Alterations of regional cerebral blood flow detected by TC 99m-HMPAO SPECT. *Arch. Neurol.* **47**, 578–584.

Watson, R.T., Valenstein, E. & Heilman, K.M. (1981): Thalamic neglect. Possible role of the medial thalamus and nucleus reticularis in behaviour. *Arch. Neurol.* **38**, 501–506.

Zimmerman, R.A., Bilaniuk, L.T., Packer, R.J., Goldberg, H.I. & Grossman, R.I. (1983): Computed tomographic arteriographic correlates in acute basal ganglionic infarction of childhood. *Neuroradiology* **24**, 241–248.

Chapter 7

Aphasic syndromes and localization of lesions in children

Philippe F. Paquier*, Hugo R. van Dongen†

Hôpital Universitaire Erasme ULB, Service de Neurologie, 808, route de Lennik, B–1070 Brussels, Belgium, and University of Antwerp (UIA), School of Medicine, Department of ENT-Surgery, B–2610 Wilrijk, Belgium; †University Hospital Rotterdam, Sophia Children's Hospital, Department of Child Neurology, dr. Molewaterplein 60, NL–3015 GJ Rotterdam, The Netherlands

Summary

The study of acquired childhood aphasia (ACA) has made significant progress in the past 20 years. From highlighting fundamental differences between childhood and adulthood aphasia for more than a century, it has evolved since the late 1970s towards an acknowledgement of fundamental similarities between both (Woods, 1985b). Regarding the clinical picture, it is clear that the traditional view asserting the universality of nonfluency in ACA is no longer tenable. Other types of semiological pictures co-exist besides the classically reported nonfluent type. They may even correspond to syndromes which infrequently occur in adults. Moreover, neuroradiological data support the current opinion that in children, lesion location and clinical picture are interrelated in a similar manner as in adults.

Introduction

Delineation and characteristics of aphasia

In a comprehensive review of aphasic syndromes, Damasio (1992) defines aphasia as 'a disturbance of the comprehension and formulation of language caused by dysfunction in specific brain regions'. Adult aphasics, he continues, 'can no longer accurately convert the sequences of non-verbal mental representations that constitute thought into the symbols and grammatical organization that constitute language [p. 531]'. Conversely, the generation of mental representations corresponding to a sentence that is heard or seen, is also defective in aphasia. Damasio (1992) further emphasizes that aphasia is neither a disorder of perception (deafness, for instance, does not hinder language comprehension through other channels than the auditory one) nor a motor speech disorder (dysarthria, for instance, leaves language formulation intact). Finally, aphasia is not a disorder of the basic thought processes such as those occurring in schizophrenia. Aphasia can result from any neurological lesion that affects the cerebral hemispheres, provided that language-related areas are involved: vascular diseases, traumatic head injuries, tumours, infectious diseases, degenerative or toxic processes, convulsive disorders. The lesions that cause aphasia in right and left-handers are usually located in the left cerebral hemisphere (Damasio, 1992; Kirshner, 1995).

Table 1. Main aphasia syndromes according to traditional aphasiology (Damasio, 1992; Kirshner, 1995)

Type of aphasia	Spontaneous speech	Auditory Comprehension	Repetition	Site of lesion (left hemisphere)
Global aphasia	Nonfluent, scant, stereotyped utterances	Impaired	Impaired	Large perisylvian or separate anterior and posterior damage
Broca's aphasia	Nonfluent, poorly articulated, dysprosodic, agrammatic	Largely preserved	Impaired	Frontal (inferior and posterior)
Transcortical motor aphasia	Nonfluent, decreased speech initiation, effortful, perseverative, stutterlike, poorly articulated	Largely preserved	Largely preserved	Anterior or superior to Broca's area (ACA-ACM watershed area)
Mixed transcortical aphasia	Nonfluent, scant, stereotyped utterances, echolalic	Impaired	Largely preserved	Massive hemispheric damage with sparing of perisylvian area
Wernicke's aphasia	Fluent, abundant, well articulated, melodic, paraphasic, paragrammatic*	Impaired	Impaired	Temporal (superior and posterior)
Transcortical sensory aphasia	Fluent, paraphasic, well articulated, melodic, echolalic	Impaired	Largely preserved	Posterior or inferior to Wernicke's area (ACM-ACP watershed area)
Conduction aphasia	Fluent, phonemic paraphasias, well articulated, melodic, conduites d'approche	Largely preserved	Impaired	Supramarginal gyrus, insula, arcuate fasciculus
Anomic aphasia	Fluent, empty, circumlocutory, well articulated, word-finding pauses, melodic	Largely preserved	Largely preserved	No specific localization

ACA = arteria cerebri anterior; ACM = arteria cerebri media; ACP = arteria cerebri posterior. *When fluent speech becomes completely incomprehensible because of excessive errors, the aphasia is termed *jargon aphasia*.

Clinical classification systems traditionally distinguish eight aphasic syndromes related to different cortical lesion localizations (Table 1). In addition, the introduction of modern neuroradiological techniques in the late 1970s and early 1980s has made it possible to relate aphasic syndromes to subcortical lesions as well. As denoted by the term 'subcortical', these syndromes are defined by the anatomy of the lesion rather than by the language characteristics, but different patterns of language difficulties have also been described (Kirshner, 1995). On the basis of their spontaneous speech characteristics, aphasic patients are often dichotomized according to a fluent/nonfluent division. Typically, nonfluent aphasic patients are considered to have a slow, reduced, and effortful speech. Their oral productions are poorly articulated, and lack the melodic modulation that characterizes normal speech (dysprosody). The utterances consist of short, one- to four-word phrases containing many pauses (which may outnumber the words themselves). Quality of articulation can vary as a function of the familiarity of the words in the utterances (e.g. conversational stereotypes). Some patients have a subset of well practiced words that can be normally articulated, whereas more difficult or uncommon words are distorted. Nonfluent aphasics often feature agrammatism, i.e. a disorder of syntax and morphology which Goodglass (1993) describes as follows: a reduction of the sentence to its skeleton, with relative abundance of substantives and almost invariable use of verbs in the infinitive, with suppression of grammatical morphemes and loss of grammatical differentiation of tense, gender, number, as well as of subordination. Auditory comprehension in nonfluent aphasia is relatively better preserved than oral expression, such that the patients appear to understand simple conversation. Synonyms of nonfluent aphasia are *motor aphasia* and *expressive aphasia*.

On the other hand, fluent aphasic patients typically speak effortlessly, with normal melody and articulation. Their utterances are produced without excessive pauses, at normal or even faster than normal rates, and generally contain more than four words. The output can sometimes become so excessive that the patients speak continuously unless forced to stop by the examiner, a phenomenon called 'logorrhoea' (or 'press of speech'). Word finding is often restricted so that despite the normal number of words uttered, conversation becomes circumlocutory and empty. Fluent aphasics can show paragrammatism, i.e. errors in the use of grammatical rules resulting in incorrect verb tenses, inappropriate conditional clauses, substitutions of grammatical morphemes, incoherent and aimless syntactic structures (nouns appearing in verb slots and vice versa) (Goodglass, 1993). Fluent aphasic patients often produce numerous phonemic and verbal substitutions (paraphasias). In severe cases, their productions may consist of an excessive number of paraphasic substitutions embedded in pseudo-grammatical sentences with erroneous morphemes and ill-chosen verb inflections. This unintelligible gibberish is referred to as 'jargon aphasia'. Auditory comprehension in fluent aphasia is often defective, in severe cases even for common objects names. Synonyms of fluent aphasia are *sensory aphasia* and *receptive aphasia*.

Delineation of acquired childhood aphasia

From the preceding it appears that in adults the use of the term 'aphasia' implies that language had already been acquired prior to lesion onset. In children on the contrary, the term has been used in reference to a number of language impairments attributable to both developmental and acquired disorders. Thus, congenital, developmental and acquired aphasia have been distinguished. According to Vargha-Khadem *et al.* (1985), *congenital aphasia* is a language disorder caused by early and extensive cerebral lesions in the thalamo-cortical projection system. Due to such demonstrable structural lesions, children with congenital aphasia fail to develop normal language functions (Landau *et al.*, 1960).

Following Woods (1985a), *developmental aphasia* (also called 'developmental dysphasia' or 'specific language impairment') refers to 'a level of language function that is significantly below age norms, has always been so (i.e. it has not been arrested at, nor has it declined from an earlier level) and is not adequately accounted for by general mental retardation, peripheral sensory or motor defects, severe emotional disturbance, or major environmental deprivation [p.

139].' Aram (1991) emphasizes that a frank neurological basis is not apparent in developmental aphasia. Both congenital and developmental aphasia share the common feature that the pathological process which prevents the normal development of language is already present before language skills begin to emerge.

In agreement with Hécaen (1976), we consider *acquired childhood aphasia* (ACA) to refer 'only to disturbances of language due to cerebral lesions which have occurred after language acquisition [p. 115]'. In contrast with the above mentioned types of childhood aphasia, in ACA the pathological process which compromises the functioning of language is sustained after a period of language development. Because lesions sustained after 1 year of age leave more severe language sequelae than those incurred prior to age 1 (Woods & Carey, 1979), the somewhat arbitrary demarcation for the onset of language was fixed at that age (Aram, 1991). The upper limit of language development conventionally corresponds to early adolescence (Woods, 1985b). We must keep in mind, however, that these boundaries are artificial, and one could – quite rightly – argue that language already begins to develop in the preverbal period before age 1 (Marchman et al., 1991), and further evolves throughout the entire life span (enrichment of vocabulary has no age limitation whatever).

The subject of the present chapter – in which we adhere to the above-mentioned definitions and the arbitrary limits proposed for delimiting the field of ACA – is the study of children who acquired aphasia following brain lesions sustained after onset of language development.

The traditional description of acquired childhood aphasia[*]

In contrast with the diversity of adult aphasic syndromes (Table 1), traditional neurological tenets (Benson, 1967, 1979; Geschwind, 1972; Lecours & Lhermitte, 1979) maintain that ACA is invariably characterized by a nonfluent clinical picture, the cardinal features of which were listed as follows by Brown & Hécaen (1976) (see Paquier & Van Dongen, 1996):

(a) Mutism or telegraphic speech (i.e. agrammatism) at an early age, word finding difficulties (i.e. anomia) and nonfluent sound substitutions (i.e. phonemic paraphasias) somewhat later;

(b) Articulatory disorders in the context of a nonfluent state;

(c) Rare occurrence of fluent phonemic paraphasias in conversation (as in conduction aphasia);

(d) Absence of speech flow (i.e. logorrhoea), and of verbal incoherence (i.e. semantic jargon) or within-word scrambled sound structures resulting in nonexisting words (i.e. neologistic jargon);

(e) No adult-type correspondence between comprehension loss and logorrhoeic jargon;

(f) Recovery superior to recovery in adult aphasia;

(g) At an early age, even frequency of aphasia with injury to either hemisphere.

In addition, it was claimed that the clinical picture of ACA is nonfluent at all times regardless

---

[*] The Landau–Kleffner syndrome, or acquired epileptic childhood aphasia, is not considered here because of its puzzling characteristics which appear to escape the traditional description of ACA.

of lesion location (Benson, 1967; Geschwind, 1972; Guttmann, 1942). In other words, not only would a lesion in either hemisphere be associated with a nonfluent aphasia, but the anterior versus posterior location of the lesion would not play any particular role in the clinical manifestation of the language disorder.

The modern area in the study of acquired childhood aphasia

In the late 1970s, Woods & Teuber (1978) published a study of paramount importance in which they formulated several conclusions that had the classical teaching on ACA totter upon its foundations. They were the first to remark that, in the course of time, a dramatic change had occurred in the incidence of crossed aphasia in children, i.e. aphasia with right hemisphere injury in right-handers. Considering that the presence of a hemiplegia – the outstanding neurological symptom in earlier days to infer a contralateral hemispheric lesion – does not preclude a clinically unrecognized bilateral cerebral damage, especially in those studies conducted before the advent of antibiotics, these authors showed that the incidence of crossed aphasia sharply dropped from 33 per cent of the total number of childhood aphasia before 1940, to 5 per cent (after exclusion of known left-handers) in studies undertaken after 1940, if they excluded earlier studies in which reports of diffuse brain involvement due to infectious diseases were frequent. Woods & Teuber (1978) attributed the earlier incidence of crossed aphasia in children – which had been used as evidence for early equipotentiality of both hemispheres for language – to undetected bilateral cerebral damage before the introduction of antibiotics and mass immunization programmes reducing the common occurrence of neurological complications in infectious diseases (Ford & Schaffer, 1927). Woods & Teuber's (1978) second main finding was that, in reporting an instance of jargon aphasia in a 5-year-old boy, they made clear that fluent types of aphasia could indeed be observed in children. To explain the rarity of fluent ACA in earlier studies, they suggested that in early days the suspicion of aphasia only arose when a right-sided hemiparesis or hemiplegia was found on examination. They further assumed that to include aphasic children with hemiplegia only might have biased some series towards the selection of patients with anterior lesions, the latter being mainly associated with nonfluent aphasia.

As a consequence of Woods & Teuber's (1978) seminal interpretation of the early data on ACA, a new way of thinking about ACA has emerged. Together with medical progress having made it possible to recognize fluent aphasic syndromes in an early stage of the disease, this intellectual progress has resulted in the publication of several case reports describing different fluent aphasia patterns in children (reviewed by Paquier & Van Dongen, 1996).

The fluency/nonfluency dimension in acquired childhood aphasia

Two specific aspects of the traditional description, or 'standard doctrine', of ACA are now elaborated: speech fluency and lesion location. The reason for this restrictive choice is twofold. First, the relevancy of the fluency dimension is closely related to the discussion of the different aphasic symptomatologies. Secondly, the various aphasic syndromes which have been recorded in children since 1978 are related to different lesion localizations. Other aspects of ACA such as the aetiologies, the incidence, the recovery process, and the prognosis have recently been reviewed by Dennis (1997) and Paquier & Van Dongen (1998).

Several studies already focused on the fluency dimension in adults. On the basis of a statistical analysis of spontaneous speech, Howes (1964) found a speech rate ranging from 12 to 220 words per minute (wpm) in aphasics, whereas normal control subjects uttered 110 to 175 wpm.

This implies that a number of aphasic patients speak faster than normals; these patients have been termed 'fluent' or even 'hyperfluent' aphasics (Howes & Geschwind, 1964). However, Wagenaar et al. (1975) and Kerschensteiner et al. (1972) could not demonstrate such a hyperfluent rate in their patients. The last mentioned authors investigated whether the fluency/nonfluency dimension in spontaneous speech could be confirmed by cluster analysis. They showed that – if the spontaneous utterances of a group of unselected aphasic adults was rated by using six clinical speech characteristics – this procedure yielded two distinct groups which reflect 'naturally' occurring differences in language behaviour, and which correspond to the clinical syndromes of fluent and nonfluent aphasia. Moreover, they were able to rank these characteristics according to their power of discrimination between the two groups (Table 2).

Table 2. Speech variables proposed for the evaluation of aphasic spontaneous speech, ranked according to their power of discriminating between fluent and nonfluent speech, and criteria suggested for delineating fluent from nonfluent speech (Kerschensteiner et al., 1972)

Variable	Nonfluent speech	Fluent speech
Phrase length	1–2 word phrases	> 4-word phrases
Pauses	many	nomal/few
Prosody	impaired	normal
Speech rate	0–50 wpm 51–90 wpm	> 90 wpm
Effort	marked	none
Articulation	impaired	normal

wpm = words per minute

According to Benson (1967), in adults such a distinction between nonfluent and fluent speech corresponds to an anatomical distinction between anterior and posterior hemispheric lesions. An analogous differentiation between nonfluent and fluent aphasia on the one hand, and between anterior and posterior lesion location on the other hand (see later in this chapter) would not exist in children, at least as was thought before 1978.

The heterogeneity of fluent aphasic patterns reported in children in the 1980s and 1990s, and the paucity of data on fluency measurements in children prompted us to investigate whether the pattern of speech characteristics in aphasic children is similar to the one Kerschensteiner et al. (1972) found in adults. We were able to analyse spontaneous conversational speech in 24 children with ACA (manuscript in preparation), and present preliminary findings which concern the analysis of phrase length and of speech rate.

Figures 1 and 2 display the results of the analysis of phrase length. The y-axis represents the number of children, the x-axis gives the percentages of one and two-word phrases (Fig. 1), and of more than four-word phrases (Fig. 2), with reference to the total number of sentences recorded in a sample of spontaneous speech. When looking at both figures, our preliminary findings suggest that:

(a) There exists a group of children who are predominantly uttering one or two-word phrases. In other words, in their spontaneous speech the occurrence of one or two-word phrases constitutes 50 up to 100 per cent of all sentences uttered during conversation. Phrases containing more than four words do not represent more than 30 per cent of the total number of their utterances.

Chapter 7 Aphasic syndromes and localization of lesions in children

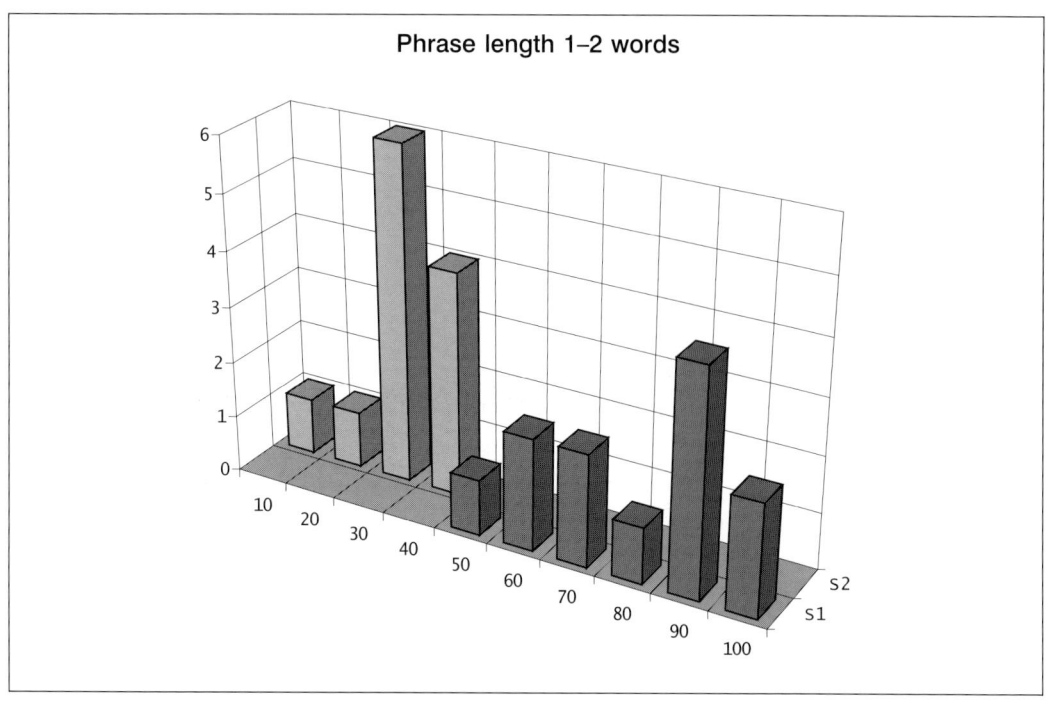

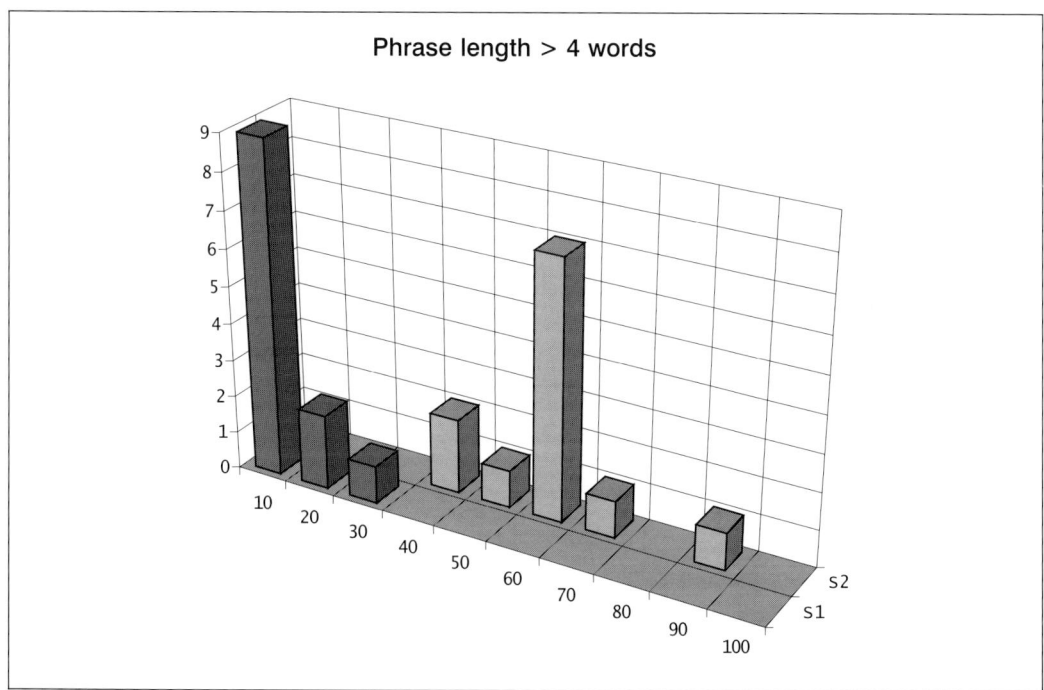

Figs. 1 & 2. Distribution of phrase length (one or two-word phrases, and > four-word phrases) in the fluent and nonfluent group. S1 (dark bars) = nonfluent group; S2 (light bars) = fluent group; values on x-axis = % one and two-word phrases, and > four-word phrases, respectively, with respect to the total number of utterances; y-axis = number of children.

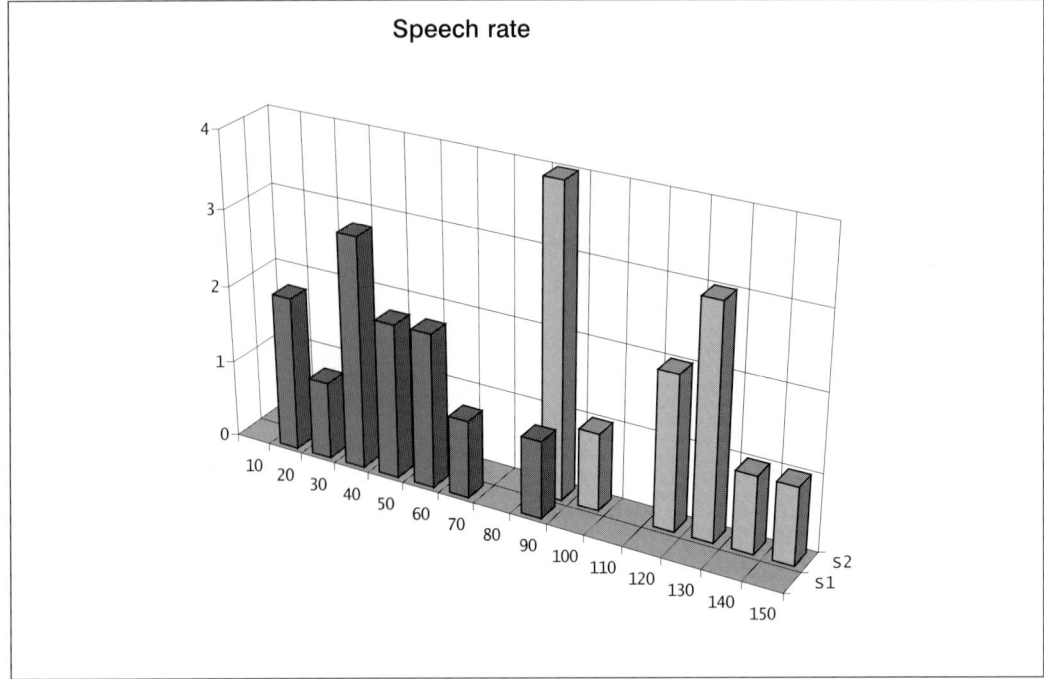

Fig. 3. Distribution of rate of speaking in the fluent and nonfluent group. S1 (dark bars) = nonfluent group; S2 (light bars) = fluent group; values on x-axis = speech rate expressed in words per minute; y-axis = number of children.

(b) There exists another group of children who use phrases longer than four words in more than 30 per cent of their utterances. These children use short phrases of one or two words in less than 40 per cent of the total number of their utterances.

In other words, our preliminary findings suggest the existence of two distinct groups, namely a group of children who speak predominantly in phrases longer than four words, and another group of children who speak mostly in phrases containing one or two words. This distinction according to phrase length seems to correspond to the values Kerschensteiner *et al.* (1972) found in adult aphasics, and which, according to these authors, differentiate between fluent and nonfluent aphasic speech.

The analysis of speech rate is even more illustrative. Figure 3 shows the speech rate expressed in words per minute on the x-axis, and the number of children in each category on the y-axis. One group of children clearly produces less than 80 wpm, whereas the other group is situated above 90 wpm. The group that utters more than 90 wpm corresponds to Kerschensteiner *et al.*'s (1972) criterium for fluent speech rate, according to their study in adult aphasics.

Consequently, our preliminary results clearly confirm the existence of a group of aphasic children who do not fit in with the standard doctrine, which claims that the clinical picture of ACA is always nonfluent. Our findings are in keeping with those reported by Van Dongen *et al.* (1994), who were able to demonstrate the existence of fluent ACA by means of an instrumental analysis of spontaneous conversational speech. Moreover, our findings are also in accordance with the still increasing number of case studies documenting a variety of different fluent clinical pictures which closely resemble the aphasic syndromes described in adults: jargon aphasia, Wernicke's aphasia, transcortical sensory aphasia, conduction aphasia, anomic aphasia, alexia without agraphia (Paquier & Van Dongen, 1996, 1998).

Localization of lesions in acquired childhood aphasia

As already seen in this chapter, traditional neurological tenets not only deny the possibility of a differentiation between fluent and nonfluent aphasia in children, but also refute any relation between the nonfluent nature of ACA and the location of the lesion within the left or right hemisphere (the standard doctrine claims that ACA frequently occurs after a right hemisphere lesion!). In a recent review of the literature, however, Paquier & Van Dongen (1996) only rarely came across a neuroradiologically well-documented case of ACA associated with a right-sided lesion. As in adults, the aphasia was caused by a left hemispheric lesion in a majority of cases. This confirms Woods & Teuber's (1978) seminal analysis of the early literature. Paquier & Van Dongen (1996) further contradicted the common belief that the clinical picture is not dependent on the location of the lesion. Reviewing the cases of fluent ACA published since 1978, they showed that, after exclusion of cases with bilateral lesions or with data too vague to allow reliable conclusions, the lesion associated with fluent aphasia was confined to the posterior brain areas in 76 per cent of the 33 children remaining for analysis (Table 3).

Table 3. Clinicoradiological correlations in fluent ACA reported since 1978 (Paquier & Van Dongen, 1996)

Type of aphasia	Number of cases	Handedness	Site of lesion
Jargon aphasia	1	R	F-T
Wernicke's aphasia	12	R	F (n = 2) T (n = 8) P (n = 1) T-P-O (n = 1)
Transcortical sensory aphasia	8	R (n = 4) L (n = 1) ? (n = 3)	F-T-P (n = 2) T (n = 1) T-P (n = 3) P (n = 1) T-O (n = 1)
Conduction aphasia	6	R	F-T-P (n = 2) T (n = 2) T-P (n = 1) P (n = 1)
Anomic aphasia	5	R	F (n = 1) T (n = 2) T-P (n = 1) P (n = 1)
Alexia without agraphia	1	R	T-O

L = left; R = right; ? = information not provided; F = frontal; T = temporal; P = parietal; O = occipital.

Consequently, this finding parallels the adult-type correlation between fluent aphasia and posterior lesion location. From another review of the literature (Paquier & Van Dongen, 1998) it appears that children who acquired a nonfluent type of aphasia (global aphasia, Broca's aphasia, transcortical motor aphasia) sustained the lesion mainly in left pre- or perirolandic areas, either subcortically or cortico-subcortically. In our preliminary reference to the series of 24 children in whom we analysed spontaneous speech fluency, the data also tend to support the above-mentioned parallel: most children displaying a fluent type of aphasia had sustained a temporo-parietal lesion, whereas the children in the nonfluent group displayed mostly fronto-temporal lesions.

Conclusions

Contrary to the traditional claim that ACA is always nonfluent irrespective of lesion location, the recent literature clearly shows that lesions in different areas of the left hemisphere can be associated with different aphasic syndromes. In most instances, the aphasic syndrome paralleled the one which would be seen in adults with a similarly located lesion. The recent data relating aphasia to a left hemisphere lesion, and the existence of fluent types of ACA in young children aged 6 or less, support the current view that in right-handed individuals, the neuronal substrate for the processing of most aspects of language is present early in life in the left hemisphere, possibly in pre-determined specific brain regions (as in adults).

Acknowledgement: Eef Poppe, MA and Frank Paemeleire, MA (Speech and Hearing Rehabilitation Centre, Ghent University Hospital, Belgium) transcribed and analysed the recordings of the 24 children of whom preliminary findings are presented in the chapter.

References

Aram, D.M. (1991): Acquired aphasia in children. In: *Acquired aphasia*, ed. M.T. Sarno, pp. 425–453. Orlando: Academic Press.

Benson, D.F. (1967): Fluency in aphasia: correlation with radioactive scan localization. *Cortex* **3**, 373–394.

Benson, D.F. (1979): *Aphasia, alexia, and agraphia*. New York: Churchill Livingstone.

Brown, J.W. & Hécaen, H. (1976): Lateralization and language representation: observations on aphasia in children, left-handers, and 'anomalous' dextrals. *Neurology* **26**, 183–189.

Damasio, A.R. (1992): Aphasia. *N. Engl. J. Med.* **326**, 531–539.

Dennis, M. (1997): Acquired disorders of language in children. In: *Behavioral neurology and neuropsychology*, eds. T.E. Feinberg & M.J. Farah, pp. 737–754. New York: McGraw-Hill.

Ford, F.R. & Schaffer, A.J. (1927): The etiology of infantile acquired hemiplegia. *Arch. Neurol. Psychiat.* **18**, 323–347.

Geschwind, N. (1972): Disorders of higher cortical function in children. *Clin. Proc. Children's Hosp. Natl. Med. Ctr.* **28**, 262–272.

Goodglass, H. (1993): *Understanding aphasia*. San Diego: Academic Press.

Guttmann, E. (1942): Aphasia in children. *Brain* **65**, 205–219.

Hécaen, H. (1976): Acquired aphasia in children and the ontogenesis of hemispheric functional specialization. *Brain Lang.* **3**, 114–134.

Howes, D. (1964): Application of the word-frequency concept to aphasia. In: *Disorders of language*, eds. A.V.S. de Reuck & M. O'Connor, pp. 47–75. London: Churchill.

Howes, D. & Geschwind, N. (1964): Quantitative studies of aphasic language. In: *Disorders of communication*, eds. D.M. Rioch & E.A. Weinstein, pp. 229–244. Baltimore: Williams and Wilkins.

Kerschensteiner, M., Poeck, K. & Brunner, E. (1972): The fluency-nonfluency dimension in the classification of aphasic speech. *Cortex* **8,** 233–247.

Kirshner, H.S. (1995): Classical aphasia syndromes. In: *Handbook of neurological speech and language disorders*, ed. H.S. Kirshner, pp. 57–89. New York: Marcel Dekker.

Landau, W.M., Goldstein, R. & Kleffner, F.R. (1960): Congenital aphasia: a clinicopathologic study. *Neurology* **10,** 915–921.

Lecours, A.R. & Lhermitte, F. (1979): Formes cliniques de l'aphasie. In: *L'aphasie*, eds. A.R. Lecours & F. Lhermitte, pp. 111–151. Paris: Flammarion Médecine-Sciences.

Marchman, V.A., Miller, R. & Bates, E.A. (1991): Babble and first words in children with focal brain injury. *Appl. Psycholinguistics* **12,** 1–22.

Paquier, P.F. & Van Dongen, H.R. (1996): Review of research on the clinical presentation of acquired childhood aphasia. *Acta Neurol. Scand.* **93,** 428–436.

Paquier, P.F. & Van Dongen, H.R. (1998): Is acquired childhood aphasia atypical? In: *Aphasia in atypical populations*, eds. P. Coppens, Y. Lebrun & A. Basso, pp. 67–115. Mahwah: Lawrence Erlbaum Associates.

Van Dongen, H.R., Paquier, P.F., Raes, J. & Creten, W.L. (1994): An analysis of spontaneous conversational speech fluency in children with acquired aphasia. *Cortex* **30,** 619–633.

Vargha-Khadem, F., Watters, G.V. & O'Gorman, A.M. (1985): Development of speech and language following bilateral frontal lesions. *Brain Lang.* **25,** 167–183.

Wagenaar, E., Snow, C. & Prins, R. (1975): Spontaneous speech of aphasic patients: a psycholinguistic analysis. *Brain Lang.* **2,** 281–303.

Woods, B.T. (1985a): Developmental dysphasia. In: *Handbook of clinical neurology. Neurobehavioural disorders*, ed. J.A.M. Frederiks, vol. 46, pp. 139–145. Amsterdam: Elsevier Science Publishers.

Woods, B.T. (1985b): Acquired aphasia in children. In: *Handbook of clinical neurology. Neurobehavioural disorders*, ed. J.A.M. Frederiks, vol. 46, pp. 147–157. Amsterdam: Elsevier Science Publishers.

Woods, B.T. & Carey, S. (1979): Language deficits after apparent clinical recovery from childhood aphasia. *Ann. Neurol.* **6,** 405–409.

Woods, B.T. & Teuber, H.L. (1978): Changing patterns of childhood aphasia. *Ann. Neurol.* **3,** 273–280.

Chapter 8

The role of the left hemisphere in processing visuospatial information

Joan Stiles* and Antigona Martinez†

Departments of Cognitive Science and Radiology,† University of California, 9500 Gilman Drive, Dept. 0515, San Diego, La Jolla, CA 92093, USA*

Summary

The traditional neuropsychological literature has emphasized a simple functional dichotomy between language and spatial cognitive processing. Specifically, language is considered to be a left hemisphere function and spatial processing a right hemisphere function. This chapter reviews data on the anatomical and functional organization of a variety of spatial processing functions, examining in each case the question of lateralization. The review of spatial processes is used as a convenient organization to structure the anatomical division between the dorsal and ventral stream processes. The first part of the chapter considers the lateralizaton of spatial processes associated with the dorsal, or 'where', system processes. The second part considers ventral, or 'what', system processes.

The role of the left hemisphere in processing visuospatial information

Traditional accounts of brain laterality typically associate the left (or dominant) hemisphere with language processing and the right (or nondominant) hemisphere with spatial processing. While there is clear evidence that, in most individuals, the left hemisphere (LH) is the principal mediator of language processing, it is becoming equally clear that it also plays an important role in many aspects of visuospatial processing. In some cases the LH appears to process spatial information in parallel with homologous systems in the right hemisphere (RH), while in other cases the left-lateralized functions are complementary to related right-lateralized functions. The purpose of this paper is to review the literature on lateralized processing for a variety of basic visuospatial processes, and in each case examine whether or to what extent the LH makes parallel or complementary contributions to the spatial information processing task.

Spatial processing encompasses a wide range of functions from object localization, to tracking a moving object, to understanding how the parts of an object combine to form an organized whole. Studies of visual system architecture have identified literally dozens of interrelated visual areas in the posterior cortices, each of which contributes to some aspect of visuospatial

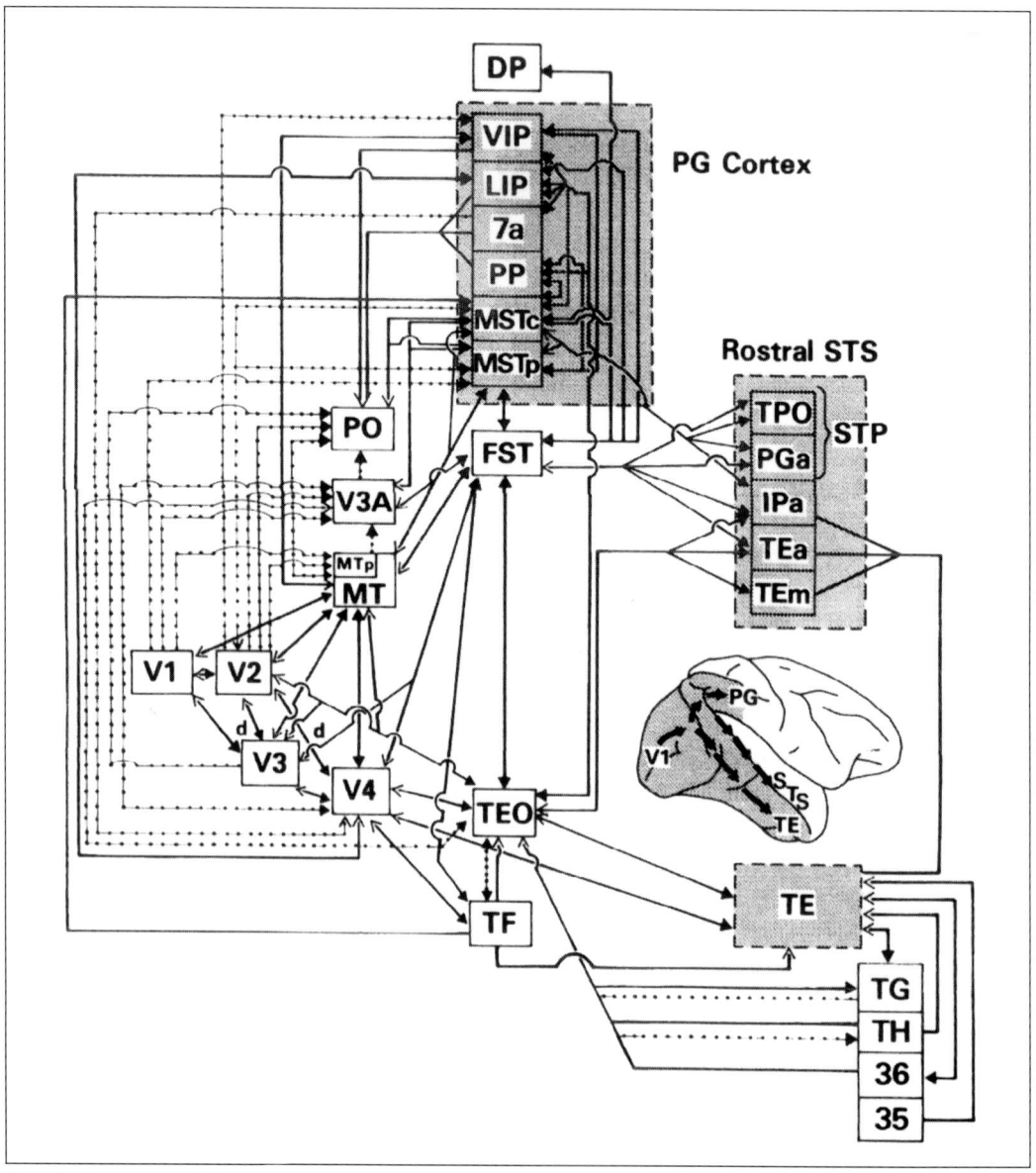

Fig. 1. Overview of the dorsal ('where') and ventral ('what') visual processing pathways. Adapted from Functional brain imaging studies of cortical mechanisms for memory, *by L. Ungerleider, 1995, Science* **270**, *770.*

processing. One very useful scheme for understanding the organization of these areas was proposed in the early 1980s by Mishkin et al. (1983). According to their proposal, the visual system can be usefully subdivided into two principal processing streams (see Fig. 1), a dorsal pathway and a ventral pathway. The dorsal pathway begins at the retina, projects via the lateral geniculate nucleus (LGN) of the thalamus to primary visual cortex, area V1. From there the pathway proceeds to areas V2 and V3, then projects dorsally to the medial (MT/V5) and medial superior (MST) regions of the temporal lobe, and then to the ventral inferior-parietal lobe (IP). The dorsal stream processes information about optic flow and other aspects of motion and about spatial location, and plays an important role in allocation of spatial attention. It has thus been described as the 'where' pathway (but also see Goodale & Milner, 1992, for discussion of the role of the inferior parietal lobe in visual control of motor output).

The ventral pathway also begins at the retina, and projects via the LGN of the thalamus to primary visual cortex, area V1. From there the pathway proceeds to areas V2 and V4, and then projects ventrally to the posterior (AIT) and anterior (PIT) regions of the inferior temporal lobe. The ventral stream processes information about visual properties of objects and patterns, and has been described as the 'what' pathway. Both the dorsal and ventral pathways project rostrally to both common and adjacent areas of the prefrontal cortex. Finally, there is substantial evidence that the two pathways are richly interconnected and at least partially overlapping (Merigan & Maunsell, 1993). This anatomical division of function provides a convenient organizational structure for discussing functional lateralization of spatial processes. The next two sections will review evidence for LH participation in the spatial functions associated with processing in the dorsal and ventral streams, respectively.

Lateralization of spatial processes associated with the dorsal stream: motion, location, and attention to space

A variety of spatial processes have been associated with activation of the dorsal visual pathway. Three of the most basic will be considered in this section: (a) perception of motion, (b) perception and memory for spatial location, and (c) spatial attention. The division into three distinct processes is somewhat artificial in that, for example, localization of an object also requires a shift in spatial attention. None-the-less, there is substantial evidence for functional and anatomical independence of key features of each process, and each provides insight to the role of the LH in basic spatial functioning. All three functions are, at least to some degree, bilaterally mediated and thus involve both LH and RH processing systems. The profiles of lateralized processing for each function will be considered.

Perception of motion

Perception of a moving object is clearly critical to our interpretation of the organization of a spatial array. Movement of elements in a visual array initiates a set of complex processes beginning at the retina and extending to target regions along the dorsal pathway. The anatomy of the motion detection system has been studied extensively in macaque monkeys (e.g. Albright, 1984; Zeki, 1978). Different features of movement are processed at different levels of the system. Motion-sensitive cells in area V1 respond to the movement of simple pattern components moving in a single direction, perpendicular to the axis of orientation of the cell's receptive field. Such 'component direction selective cells' are also common much further down the dorsal processing stream; approximately 80 per cent of cells in area V5 (also called MT) display orientation and direction specificity to simple pattern components. However, within area V5, there is a smaller population of cells that are sensitive to the motion of more complex pattern movement. These 'pattern direction sensitive cells' receive and integrate input from multiple component direction sensitive cells. These cells are thus responsive to information from a much broader extent of the visual array, and provide information about more global properties of pattern movement. Experimental lesions to area V5 result in selective deficits of complex motion perception (Cowey & Marcar, 1992a, 1992b; Newsome & Pare, 1988).

Although the data from studies of monkeys have provided an elegant and convincing model for the role of area V5 in motion processing, data on a comparable centre in humans has, until recently, been limited. Specific deficits of movement perception, or akinetopsia, in human patient populations are very interesting but extremely rare. Fortunately, recent advances in functional imaging technology have made it possible to identify profiles of activation in response to movement cues within the dorsal pathway in humans (e.g. Tootell et al., 1995; Watson et al., 1993; Zeki et al., 1991). A review of the data from an important case study of akinetopsia, and from the recent functional imaging studies in normal adults, provides persuasive evidence for a human analogue of the motion processing area V5. All of these studies indicate that perception of complex motion is bilaterally mediated within homologous anatomical regions of the RH and LH that operate symmetrically and in parallel.

Zihl et al. (1983, 1991) reported an unusual case of akinetopsia. The patient, LM, was a 43-year-old woman who developed a sinus vein thrombosis resulting in headache, vertigo, nausea, and eventually stupor. CT exam at time of hospitalization showed large bilateral lesions of the occipitoparietal cortices. Subsequent MRI analysis (Shipp et al., 1994) showed approximately symmetrical lesions in the lateral occipital gyri (Brodmann's areas 37 and 19) that extended ventrally through the region of the lateral occipital sulci (the sulci were apparently destroyed in this patient). The posterior boundary of the lesion was within 2 cm of midline on the area 18/19 border; the anterior boundary includes all of areas 19 and 37. The white matter underlying the lateral occipital cortex was destroyed, however the medial cortex within the calcarine and parieto-occipital sulci was intact. LM has normal acuity, colour vision, binocular vision and stereopsis, object perception including line bisection and orientation, face and part-whole processing (Zihl et al., 1983, 1991). Her primary deficit is a profound loss of motion perception. She describes the world as appearing in a series of snapshots. She could not see movement in depth, and thus could not judge the movement of cars or see the movement of facial features when talking to people. She had difficulty with everyday tasks involving calibration of object movement, such as that required to pour a cup of tea.

Detailed studies of motion processing in LM indicated some residual motion perception ability. While she could not see movement in depth, she could detect the vertical and horizontal movement of a spot of light presented within the central but not peripheral field, but only at very slow speeds that were well below the normal threshold. She was able to detect the drift of a moving grating, but at thresholds 20× greater than normal (Hess et al., 1989), and she could perceive the movement of random dot patterns but only in the absence of visual noise (Baker et al., 1991). In a recent Positron Emission Tomography (PET) study (Shipp et al., 1994), LM was tested with a series of moving random dot patterns. Unlike normal controls, no activation was evident in area V5 (see below for further discussion of the human analogue of V5) in either hemisphere. It had been anticipated that LM's residual motion sensitivity would be mediated by areas V1 or V2. Surprisingly there was no evidence of functional activation to motion stimuli in either of these early visual cortical areas. This finding suggests that activation of areas V1 and V2 in response to complex pattern movement requires feedback from area V5. Rather, LM showed unusually enhanced activation in area V3 and in the superior parietal cortex (area 7). Finally, a recent series of case studies examining the effects of *unilateral* injury to V5, suggests that motion perception in the visual field contralateral to the side of the lesion is impaired in ways that mirror LM's bilateral impairment (Schenk & Zihl, 1997).

In the past decade, studies using PET and functional Magnetic Resonance Imaging (fMRI) have greatly enhanced our understanding of motion perception in humans. Drawing upon evidence from earlier monkey work, a number of investigators postulated that functionally dissociable regions in human cortex for motion perception could be identified. In an elegant series of studies, Zeki and his colleagues (Watson *et al.*, 1993; Zeki *et al.*, 1991) mapped a region of cortex which appears to be a principal centre for complex movement processing, and is the anatomical equivalent of area V5 in macaque. Subjects were presented with moving and stationary displays consisting of randomly placed squares on a white background. Activation areas associated with perception of movement were identified bilaterally at the confluence of temporal, parietal, and occipital cortices situated laterally on the cortical convexity (Brodmann's areas 19 and 37). The anatomical location of the motion area has been confirmed in subsequent studies using fMRI (Tootell *et al.*, 1995). Individual variation in exact anatomical location of peak intensity is as great as 27 mm in the left hemisphere and 18 mm in the right hemisphere, but the degree of overlap in the functional areas is impressive (Watson *et al.*, 1993).

In summary, data from both monkey and human studies convincingly identify a bilateral motion perception centre located in area V5 of the dorsal visual pathway. As demonstrated by difficulties encountered by patient LM, motion perception is a critical aspect of visuospatial processing that allows for the tracking of an object through space. The motion perception system is clearly represented bilaterally, with equal contributions from the right and left hemisphere visual pathways. The RH and LH centres make symmetrical and parallel contributions to the perception of complex movement.

Perception and memory of spatial location

Another important aspect of spatial processing involves perception of and memory for the location of objects in a spatial array. This section reviews data on profiles of brain activation associated with tasks in which subjects were required either to compare directly the location of elements in two perceptually available visual displays, or to hold in memory a specific target location.

Haxby & colleagues (Haxby *et al.*, 1991, 1994) have used functional imaging techniques to examine brain activation profiles in normal adult subjects on tasks requiring them to compare the location of objects in two visually presented arrays. The judgement tasks were relatively difficult ones in which subjects compared the relative location of an internally positioned object (an abstract pattern or a face) within a set of concentric rectangles. The use of appropriate control tasks and image subtraction techniques allowed the investigators to isolate specific patterns of activation associated with processing of object location. Both right and left hemisphere sites of activation were identified. In the most posterior brain regions, areas of extrastriate cortex were activated bilaterally; these included the calcarine, medial, and lateral areas of the occipital lobe. These areas are presumed to be involved in early visual processing and are typically activated on a wide array of visual processing tasks. In addition, the dorsolateral occipital (area 19) and the posterior superior parietal areas, extending rostrally to the intraparietal sulcus (area 7), were also activated bilaterally. These areas are considered to be critical to processing of location information. Finally, the dorsal lateral prefrontal cortex (area 6) was activated unilaterally on the right. This activation may be related to spatial memory demands (see below) or to eye-movement.

Spatial working memory has been a recent focus of functional imaging. Smith, Jonides & colleagues have systematically examined the activation profiles associated with tasks of spatial working memory (Jonides *et al.*, 1993; Smith *et al.*, 1995, 1996). In these studies, subjects were given a series of trials in which they were required to remember the location of a briefly presented target. The patterns of brain activation on these tasks are consistent with those reported by Haxby, but show both greater overall right lateralization and more extensive frontal activation. The primary areas of activation on the spatial memory task were right occipital (area 19), right and left parietal (area 40), right premotor (area 6), right dorsolateral prefrontal (area 47), right prefrontal (area 46), and the anterior cingulate.

Haxby (Haxby et al., 1994) has explicitly compared the patterns on his spatial perception tasks and the spatial memory tasks reported by Jonides. The two sets of tasks activated a number of common, or at least overlapping, areas. Haxby reported that the dorsolateral occipital areas identified in the two studies lie approximately 9 mm apart, the superior parietal areas are 11 mm apart and also within an activation area reported by Corbetta et al. (1993) for spatial attention tasks, and the prefrontal areas are 11 mm apart and again are consistent with areas of activation reported by Corbetta. Even with this overlap, a major distinction between the two studies, of course, consists in a marked difference in the profiles of lateralization. The spatial perception sites are all bilaterally activated, whereas two of the sites activated during the spatial memory task (occipital and frontal) are right lateralized. Furthermore, the activation profiles for the LH and RH parietal sites were not symmetrical on spatial memory tasks. Activation in the RH was greater than activation in the LH. Further, left parietal activation was not observed in all versions of the spatial memory task. Rather, it was seen only on more difficult variants suggesting that the left parietal centre may have been recruited only under conditions of enhanced task demands. Thus memory for spatial location appears to be more RH lateralized than perception of spatial location.

Spatial attention

A closely related line of investigation focuses on the neural systems associated with *attention* to different locations in space. In contrast to the work examining profiles of brain activity when subjects are required to directly perceive or remember the location of an object in space, spatial attention tasks investigate the brain systems activated when subjects are asked to shift their attention to different locations in the spatial array. The ability to shift attention to different spatial locations is one part of the larger attentional system involving widely distributed brain areas. Review of the full literature on attention is well beyond the scope of this chapter. This section will focus more narrowly on those aspects of the attention system involved in shifting attention in space.

Any visual scene presents a complex array of features and objects. To make sense of the visual world it is necessary to identify and integrate the perceived elements, but to do that it is also necessary to focus attention on the various elements in the array in sequence. Patients with a rare disorder known as Balint's syndrome illustrate the importance of being able to shift attention between elements in the array. Balint's syndrome is a complex disorder typically asssociated with large bilateral parietal lesions; it involves a variety of specific impairments including gaze and fixation disorders, optic ataxia, and disturbances of visual attention (Heilman & Valenstein, 1993). The visual attentional impairment is particularly striking. These patients appear to be unable to focus on more than one feature of a visual display or to shift their attention readily between items. The disorder can be extreme. For example, Rafal (Rafal & Robertson, 1995) reported the case of a woman who could not look at someone *and* tell if she was wearing glasses, though she could identify the face and the glasses if either were presented separately.

There is considerable evidence that the posterior parietal lobes play a crucial role in the ability to shift attention to different spatial locations (Hillyard & Anllo-Vento, 1998; Ivry & Robertson, 1998; Posner, 1980; Posner et al., 1984; Robertson, 1992). Posner's (Posner, 1980; Posner & Petersen, 1990) model of the attention system involves an interconnected network of structures that modulate and control different aspects of attention. According to Posner, the parietal lobes play an essential role in disengaging attention from one location and allowing a shift of attention to another location. The standard task used to demonstrate covert attention shifts uses reaction time to measure changes in performance under both valid and invalid attentional cueing conditions.

In one simple version of this task, subjects are seated in front of a computer monitor and instructed to fixate, continuously, a point located centrally between two identical, flanking squares. After some fixed period, a visual cue is presented either centrally (e.g. an arrow pointing right or left) or peripherally (e.g. one box brightens briefly), and soon after a target appears very briefly in one of the boxes. The subject's task is to respond as soon as the target is detected. The critical variable in these experiments is the validity of the cue. On most trials (75–80 per cent) the cue is 'valid' and the target appears in the box indicated by the cue. On the remaining trials, the cue is 'invalid'. That is, the target appears in the opposite box. The question is, then, does cueing serve to shift attention (covertly) to the cued location? If so, it should take less time to report the presence of the target when the cue is valid (because the location of the target and attention are coincident), than when the cue is invalid (because it takes time to shift attention to the new location). At this point, literally hundreds of experiments have demonstrated the efficacy of this task in assessing shifts of spatial attention in normal populations. In addition, tasks of this sort have proven extremely useful in the study of patients diagnosed with disorders of spatial attention.

Using a variant of the attentional cueing task, Corbetta (Corbetta, 1998; Corbetta et al., 1993) examined patterns of brain activation to shifts of attention within the right and left visual fields (RVF, LVF). A major focus of this study was the profiles of activation within right and left parietal regions. The results of this study confirmed earlier reports from both human and animal work on the role of the parietal lobes in shifting spatial attention. Significant foci of brain activation were observed in both left and right superior parietal regions. However, the patterns of activation to stimuli presented to the RVF and LVF were not symmetrical across the hemispheres. Presentation of targets to the LVF produced significantly more activation in the RH than the LH, while presentation of targets to the RVF produced significant levels of activation in both the RH and LH. Furthermore, distinct activation sites for RVF and LVF targets were identified within the right superior parietal region, thus suggesting that different brain regions within the RH are responsible for processing information from the two sides of space. These data suggest that while shifts of attention to the left side of space are mediated predominantly by the RH, attention to the left side of space is bilaterally mediated.

A similar pattern of parietal activation was obtained on a second, related spatial attention task, visual search. Visual search tasks require subjects to detect a target in an array of distractors. For some kinds of single features of stimuli, such as colour or shape, target detection is immediate and does not require a search for the target through the visual array (Treisman & Gelade, 1980). For more complex stimuli (conjunction stimuli) a serial search through the array is necessary to find the target. The process of visual search requires the subject to repeatedly shift attention from one item to the next, a process similar to that required in the visual cueing task. Corbetta (Corbetta et al., 1995) measured patterns of brain activation using PET while subjects were engaged in a series of visual search tasks. During feature searches, little superior parietal activation was observed. However, considerable parietal activation was found during the conjunction search task. Activation was stronger in the RH than the LH. Comparison of the specific anatomical activation sites observed on the visual search task with those obtained on the cued attention task revealed a very close correspondence in patterns of parietal activation across the two tasks. This convergence of findings provides strong evidence for the role of the superior parietal lobes in shifting visual attention, and for the asymmetrical contributions of the two hemispheres in this type of processing.

Hemispatial neglect is an attentional disorder frequently observed following unilateral parietal injury. In severe cases, hemispatial neglect patients appear to be unaware of objects and events in the visual hemispace contralateral to their lesion (Heilman & Valenstein, 1993). They may eat only half the food on their plate, fail to comb half of their hair, and on simple paper and pencil copying task they fail to reproduce half of the model form. Impairments associated with neglect cannot be accounted for by sensory deficits. Indeed, the disruption experienced by neglect patients may be more devastating than those experienced by patients with visual sensory deficits (McFie et al., 1950). There is evidence that the attentional disorder may extend beyond the immediate, perceptually available environment, and may include the patient's representation of space (e.g. Bisiach & Luzzatti, 1978). In many patients a milder form of hemispatial inattention known as extinction is evident. These patients appear to be able to attend to the contralesional field if there are no distractors in the ipsilesional field. For example, a patient may be able to identify an object presented singly to either the right or left visual field, but when two objects are presented simultaneously, one to each field, the patient fails to identify the object in the contralesional field. A number of theories have been proposed to account for neglect disorders and the debates are far from resolved. However, complete discussion of these theories is well beyond the scope of this chapter. Instead, the focus will be on data related to impairment in the ability to shift visual attention evident in many neglect patients.

Rafal (1994) has suggested that the neglect syndrome can be 'fractionated' into a number of components, and the different components are associated with injury to different brain systems. While mild forms of neglect are apparent with injury to either right or left hemisphere brain systems, severe cases of neglect are most common with right hemisphere, specifically right temporoparietal, injury (Albert, 1973; Gainotti et al., 1972; Heilman & Valenstein, 1993; Vallar, 1993). Heilman & Van Den Abell (1980) proposed that the asymmetrical distribution of disorders related to spatial inattention may be associated with differences in the receptive properties of cells in right and left parietal cortex (also see Mesulam, 1981). Specifically, the RH has a larger proportion of cells with bilateral receptive fields than the left. While the receptive field hypothesis, *per se*, has not been specifically tested, recent functional imaging studies, such as those by Corbetta et al. (1993) discussed earlier, support the idea that attention to the visual fields may not be symmetrically distributed across the hemispheres. Moreover, lesions localized to the individual regions identified by Corbetta would lead to the profile of deficits typically reported among neglect patients. Specifically lesions to the right parietal lobe would impair attention to information in both the RVF and LVF, but since the left hemisphere is undamaged, a system for processing information in the RVF would remain intact. Lesions to the left parietal lobe would impair processing of information in the RVF, but since the RH can process information from both fields, only subtle deficits are noted.

One important distinction that has been made with regard to the distribution of attention is whether attention is object-based or space-based (Driver & Mattingley, 1995; Egly et al., 1994a, 1994b; Kanwisher & Driver, 1992). Although there is a large body of data from patients with hemispatial neglect suggesting that the observed disorders derive from inattention to the contralateral side of space, there is emerging evidence that, at for least some patients, the attentional deficit may 'travel' with the movement of the attended object. Tipper & Behrmann (1996) and Behrmann & Tipper (1994) tested patients with left neglect on a task that required them to detect a target appearing on either the left or right side of a 'barbell' shaped frame. In these studies, the frame was presented at the beginning of a trial, then, the frame either remained stationary or rotated slowly 180° such that the two sides of the barbell were reversed. Finally, the target appeared. In the stationary frame conditions, left neglect patients showed the typically impaired responses to targets presented on the left side of the frame. However, on trials when the frame rotated performance was impaired when targets appeared on the right side of the frame. When the line connecting the two sides of the barbell was eliminated, the effect of rotation on target identification was eliminated. This finding suggests that, at least for these tasks, the distribution of attention, and thus the deficit, was centred on the object rather than on the spatial location *per se*.

A study by Egly *et al.* (1994a) of patients with either left or right neglect investigated another issue related to the distinction between object-centred and space-centred attention. They examined patients' ability to shift attention either between spatial locations or between objects. Their results suggest that there may be lateralized differences in these two functions. Subjects were shown displays consisting of two long rectangular bars, one positioned on either side of a central fixation point. The bars were either arranged vertically, such that one bar was located in the right visual field and the other in the left, or they were arranged horizontally such that one was in the upper field and the other in the lower. The patients' task was to press a button when they detected a target (i.e. when an end of one of the bars whitened). The target could appear on any one of the four ends and it was preceded by a cue that was valid 75 per cent of the time and invalid 25 per cent of the time. Invalid cues always appeared in a location immediately opposite the target (i.e. they never appeared along a diagonal); on half of the trials invalid cues appeared on the same rectangle as the target and on the other half they appeared on the other rectangle. Thus, half of these trials required a shift of attention to *only* a new spatial location, and the other half required a shift to *both* a new spatial location and a new object. As in other studies, both the RH and the LH patients showed overall impairment when targets presented to the contralesional field were invalidly cued, thus reflecting an impairment in the ability to shift attention to alternate spatial locations. However, the crucial finding from this study concerned trials on which the target and invalid cue appeared in either the same or different rectangle, that is whether or not the trial required a shift of object-centred attention. For targets presented to the contralesional field (and cues to the ipsilesional field), patients with LH lesions were more impaired than patients with RH lesions when the invalid cue and target appeared in separate rectangles. Thus, in addition to impairment in their ability to shift between spatial locations (indicated by the relative slowing of responses to all targets in the contralesional field), the patients with LH injury also showed specific and pronounced deficits in shifting attention between objects in the visual array. This study suggests that while both hemispheres play a role in shifting attention to spatial location, the LH may play a unique role in shifting attention between objects in the visual array.

Converging evidence for the separate role of the LH hemisphere in shifting attention between objects was reported by Egly *et al.* (1994b) in a case study of a commisurotomy patient. Finally, Egly *et al.* suggest that the kind of profound visual attention disorder like that described above in the case of the woman with Balint's syndrome who could not tell if someone was wearing

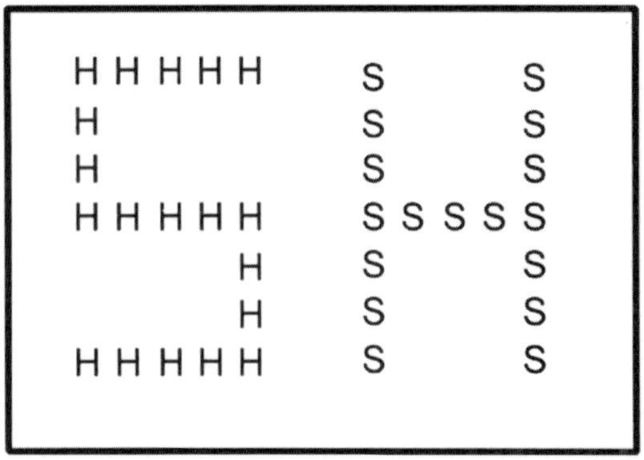

```
H H H H H      S           S
H              S           S
H              S           S
H H H H H      S S S S S
          H        S          S
          H        S          S
H H H H H      S           S
```

Fig. 2. Stimuli used in the global-local processing task.

glasses, may be accounted for by simultaneous dysfunction of object-centred and space-centred attention systems.

The data on selective visual attention present a complex mix of findings with regard to lateralization of spatial function. It is clear that both the RH and LH play important roles in mediating this aspect of visual attention. Both participate in shifting attention in the contralateral visual field. The RH appears to represent both the contralateral and ipsilateral fields, a finding that may help to explain the ubiquitous findings of asymmetrical impairment of attention following unilateral parietal brain injury. Finally, studies of object-centred attention suggest an additional, and perhaps unique, role for the LH in shifting spatial attention between objects in an array.

Lateralization of spatial processes associated with the ventral stream: understanding parts and wholes and how they go together

The relationship between 'parts' and 'wholes' has been a central issue in the study of visual perception for many years. Normal observers can easily direct attention to emphasize perception of the trees (parts) or the forest (wholes), even though these occur at different spatial scales. This ability to properly relate parts and wholes to one another is a crucial aspect of visual perception and, accordingly, has generated an extensive body of literature. Research concerning how a visual scene is segmented into its component parts and how these are then organized into a coherent whole (defined as spatial analytical, or global/local, processing), has centred around two opposing views. At one extreme is the notion that perception of the overall scene is built up from an initial analysis of the parts. The other extreme view, proposed initially by the gestalt psychologists (Koffka, 1935), is that the overall, or global, configuration of the scene is perceived first and that information about the individual parts is only subsequently extracted (see Robertson, 1986 for a review). Both of these extreme versions predict a strict order of processing. In the first, the whole cannot be perceived until the parts have been analysed and in the latter the whole must be analysed first in order to perceive the parts.

The part-whole distinction has recently been replaced with the concept of hierarchical organization. Hierarchical organization refers to the notion that perceived objects contain many levels of embedded structure. The position of an object within a hierarchical structure defines its degree of 'globalness' or 'localness'. Objects at the top of the hierarchy are more global than those lower in the hierarchy. For instance, the small letters of Fig. 2 occupy the local level of the form, whereas the large letters (e.g. the overall configuration), is at the global level. Parts and wholes, therefore, are defined by the position they occupy in the hierarchy of levels.

The human brain contains attentional and perceptual mechanisms that bind objects hierarchically and yet keeps those same objects perceptually separate. Perception of the global features of an object or visual scene is thought to be associated with a mechanism differentially biased towards the RH, whereas the LH appears to show a bias for processing information about local features or details. Studies involving adult subjects with unilateral focal brain lesions (e.g. Delis et al., 1986; Lamb et al., 1989; Robertson & Lamb, 1991; Robertson et al., 1988) have indeed shown that the side and site of brain damage disrupts global/local processing ability in different ways. For example, patient groups with lesions centred in the left posterior superior temporal gyrus (STG) have an increased global advantage (i.e. they are worse at processing the local level of a hierarchical stimulus array) relative to normals, while lesions in homologous regions of the RH are associated with a *decreased* global advantage. It is worth noting that this same pattern of hemispheric functional lateralization is observed following complete resection of the corpus callosum (i.e. 'split-brain') (Robertson et al., 1993).

Consistent with the neuropsychological literature, visual half-field (hemifield) studies with normals (Martin, 1979; Sergent, 1982) have revealed asymmetrical performance when subjects are asked to identify global and local level targets presented unilaterally to either the LVF or RVF. Sergent (1982) suggested that this hemispheric asymmetry in global/local processing was not due to differences in early (primary) visual functioning. Rather, she suggested that the hemispheres differed in terms of higher-order perceptual processes that differentially emphasized processing of lower spatial frequencies in the RH and higher spatial frequencies in the LH. In accordance with this view, experiments using sinusoidal gratings containing a single spatial frequency and appearing in the RVF or LVF, have shown that low spatial frequencies are responded to faster in the RVF than LVF and high spatial frequencies are responded to faster in the LVF than RVF (Kitterle & Selig, 1991). This pattern of hemispheric lateralization as a function of attention to spatial frequency is also observed electrophysiologically. In a recent study, Martinez et al. (1997a) recorded event-related potentials (ERPs) to sinusoidal gratings of either high or low spatial frequency content. Selection of both attended frequencies was indexed by a slow negativity (*selection negativity*, SN) broadly distributed bilaterally over the occipital scalp. The SN elicited by low spatial frequencies had a larger amplitude over the right hemisphere at the most lateral electrode sites whereas the SN associated with selection of high spatial frequency showed greater amplitude over lateral left hemisphere scalp sites.

The relationship between spatial frequency and identification of global and local levels of complex hierarchical stimuli has been the focus of several studies. Shulman et al. (1986) adapted subjects to either high or low spatial frequency gratings followed by presentation of hierarchical stimulus patterns. Prior adaptation to low spatial frequencies slowed identification of global level targets, whereas adaptation to high spatial frequencies impaired local level target detection. This asymmetry, however, is thought to be based on the *relative* spatial frequency content of the stimuli that are used and not on their absolute frequency (Lamb et al., 1990). Further support for the strong relationship between global/local identification and spatial frequency comes from studies showing that reaction time advantages for identifying global-level targets are abolished when stimuli are filtered such that all low spatial frequencies are removed from the display (i.e. high-pass filtering) (Badcock et al., 1990; Hughes et al., 1990). This effect is obtained even though the hierarchical structure of the stimulus remains intact and perceptually salient. Ivry & Robertson (1998) have argued that it is not the sensory representations of spatial frequencies that are lateralized but rather the cerebral mechanisms associated with spatial frequency filtering operations. Accordingly, these authors suggest that it is these filtering operations that are impaired with selective damage to the posterior STG. For instance, injury to RH regions results in a relative inability to detect global level information because the RH's low-pass filter is impaired. Conversely, in this case an advantage toward local level identification is observed due to the LH's intact high-pass filter.

Rather than suggesting a strict dichotomous functional separation between the hemispheres, the

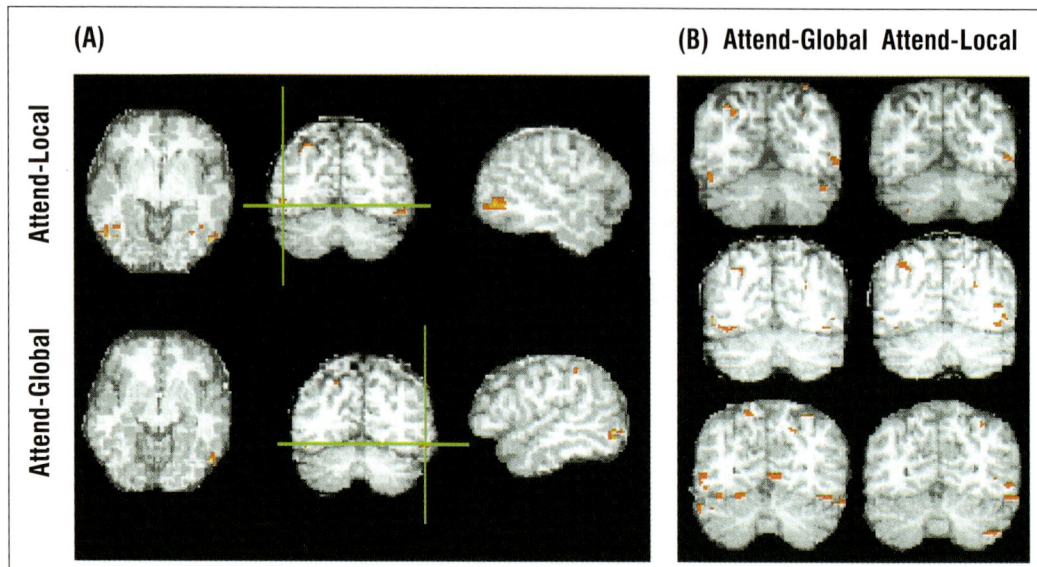

Fig. 3. (A) Activation profile of a single subject, seen in three planes. The green lines depict the position of the horizontal and lateral views. Significantly correlated voxels are shown on a red to yellow scale, voxels with highest correlation coefficient values are in yellow. The LH is on the right. (B) Activation profiles for three additional subjects in the acquired coronal plane (slice 2). Reprinted from Hemispheric asymmetries in global and local processing: evidence from fMRI, *by A. Martinez, P. Moses, L. Frank, R. Buxton, E. Wong & J. Stiles, 1997, NeuroReport 8, 1687.*

available data suggests that the observed asymmetries are due to differences in the *degree* of processing ability of the LH and RH. A recent functional magnetic resonance imaging (fMRI) study from our laboratory (Martinez *et al.*, 1997) suggests this may be the case with respect to the reported hemispheric asymmetries in global/local processing. In our study of normal adults, change in haemodynamic response, specifically blood oxygenation levels as measured by functional MRI, was used to investigate the anatomical location and magnitude of hemispheric asymmetry associated with processing hierarchical stimuli. Although it is quite likely that multiple brain regions interact to produce the behavioural profiles associated with segmentation and integration of hierarchical arrays, we focused our investigation on the role of the temporal lobes. Regions encompassed by the posterior temporal lobes (including inferior-temporal and fusiform gyri) have been identified in animal (e.g. Desimone *et al.*, 1984; Tanaka *et al.*, 1991), and in human neuroimaging studies (Haxby *et al.*, 1991; Malach *et al.*, 1995) as crucial for identifying object shape and features. Ten right-handed adults participated in the fMRI study. During the scanning session, subjects viewed centrally presented hierarchical stimuli and directed their attention to either the global or local level of the pattern in order to detect infrequent target stimuli. During one scan, subjects attended to the global shapes and ignored the local elements; during a second scan they attended the local elements and ignored the global configuration.

To analyse the fMRI data, activation in previously specified regions of interest (ROIs) in the right and left hemispheres were compared under the globally- and locally-directed conditions. The patterns of functional activation within occipitotemporal regions of the LH and RH reflected asymmetrical processing of global and local levels of pattern structure. Specifically,

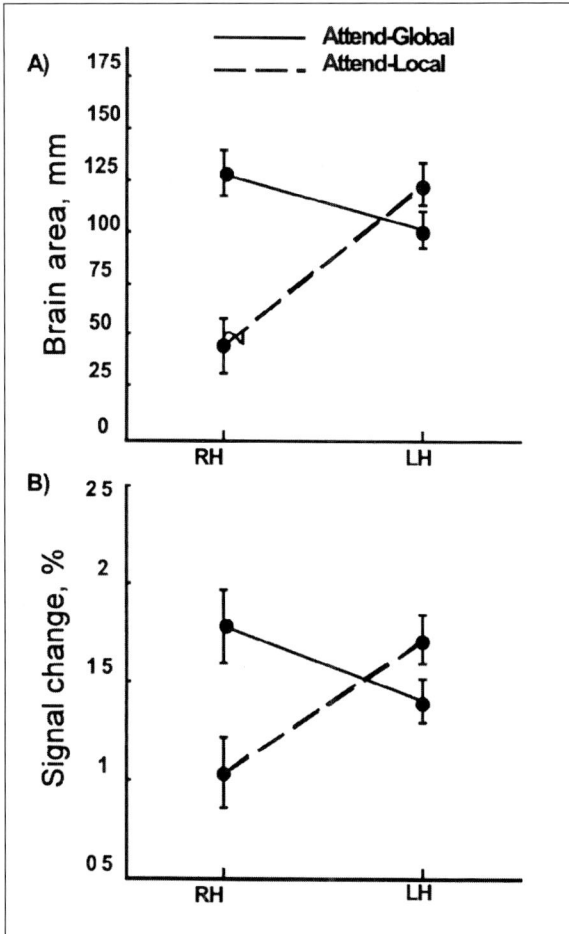

Fig. 4. Functional activation levels under attend-global and attend-local processing condition. The dependent measure in (A) is a volume measure indexing activation and in (B) it is an intensity measure indexing percentage signal change.

activation was significantly greater in the RH during the attend-global task than during attend-local, whereas the reverse was true for LH activation (see Fig. 3). Additionally, though RH activation was significantly attenuated or completely absent while subjects directed their attention to the local level, activation in the LH was observed during *both* attention conditions, with a trend for greater activation during the locally-directed condition.

These imaging results map well with previous behavioural studies from our laboratory in which hierarchical stimuli were presented either centrally, to the LVF, or to the RVF while subjects focused on a single level of structure. The increased area of activation observed in the fMRI experiment, was associated with faster reaction times (RTs) in the behavioural hemifield task. That is, RTs to stimuli appearing in the LVF/RH were fastest when subjects were directed to attend to the global level but RTs to stimuli presented to the RVF/LH were roughly equivalent regardless of which level was attended (although subjects were marginally faster to local targets). Figure 4 shows mean RTs to stimuli presented to the LVF and RVF under both task conditions, and fMRI activation profiles (measured as mean percentage signal change and accompanying activated brain area), under attend-global and attend-local conditions in right and left hemisphere ROIs.

The fMRI and RT data provide robust, consistent profiles of hemispheric differences for processing global and local pattern information. Based upon these findings, it appears that global information is processed with almost equal efficiency by both hemispheres, while local information is processed faster by the LH. Although the profiles do not indicate the strong double dissociation suggested from studies of adult lesion patients, the patterns of data are nevertheless quite consistent and indicate a bias within each hemisphere for processing different kinds of information. Consistent with other studies of global/local processing, a clear advantage for global input was observed within the RH. The dissociation within the LH was somewhat weaker, but followed the pattern of enhanced local level processing reported elsewhere. Furthermore, the profiles of activation for both RH and LH are consistent with data from our own hemifield RT task. These data suggest that while the RH demonstrates a marked global processing bias, the LH effectively processes information from both levels of pattern structure demonstrating a much less pronounced local level bias.

Summary and conclusions

This chapter reviewed findings from a large number of studies all focused on some aspect of spatial information processing. The specific goal was to examine the role of the LH in processing spatial information. The review was not intended to be a comprehensive survey of all facets of spatial information processing. Rather, it was designed to focus on several major spatial processing systems within both the dorsal and ventral visual pathways, and to use data on the anatomical organization and behavioural functioning of those systems to emphasize the bilateral organization of spatial processing in the human brain.

To say a system is bilaterally organized does not necessarily imply that it is symmetrically organized. The data presented in this chapter make this point clearly. For some processing systems reviewed here, the RH and LH contribute equally and symmetrically to the processing task. That is, they are symmetrical. The motion detection system in area V5 provides a good example of such a system. For other systems, the two hemispheres make quite different and complementary contributions. The differential role of the left and right posterior temporal lobes in global-local processing is an illustration of a complementary system. In still other cases, the LH participates in processing but plays a nondominant or nonexclusive role. The role of the LH in shifting spatial attention is an example of such a system. What is common to all of these organizational examples is that there is an essential role for the LH in each of the spatial processing systems reviewed. The old dichotomy simply does not apply. While the LH may in fact be dominant for language functioning, it also plays a significant and complex role in processing of spatial information.

References

Albert, M.D. (1973): A simple test of visual neglect. *Neurology* **23,** 658–664.

Albright, T.D. (1984): Direction and orientation selectivity of neurons in visual area MT of the macaque. *J. Neurophysiol.* **52,** 1106–1130.

Badcock, J.C., Whitworth, F.A., Badcock, D.R. & Lovegrove, W.J. (1990): Low-frequency filtering and the processing of local-global stimuli. *Perception* **19,** 617–629.

Baker Jr., C.L., Hess, R.F. & Zihl, J. (1991): Residual motion perception in a 'motion-blind' patient, assessed with limited-lifetime random dot stimuli. *J. Neurosci.* **11,** 454–461.

Behrmann, M. & Tipper, S.P. (1994): Object-based attentional mechanisms: evidence from patients with unilateral neglect. In: *Attention and performance 15: conscious and nonconscious information processing,* Attention and performance series, eds. C. Umilta & M. Moscovitch, pp. 351–375. Cambridge, MA: MIT Press.

Bisiach, E. & Luzzatti, C. (1978): Unilateral neglect of representational space. *Cortex* **14,** 129–133.

Corbetta, M. (1998): Frontoparietal cortical networks for directing attention and the eye to visual locations: identical, independent, or overlapping neural systems? *Proc. Nat. Acad. Sci. USA* **95,** 831–838.

Corbetta, M., Miezin, F.M., Shulman, G.L. & Petersen, S.E. (1993): A PET study of visuospatial attention. *J. Neurosci.* **13,** 1202–1226.

Corbetta, M., Shulman, G.L., Miezin, F.M. & Petersen, S.E. (1995): Superior parietal cortex activation during spatial attention shifts and visual feature conjunction. *Science* **270,** 802–805.

Cowey, A. & Marcar, V.L. (1992a): The effect of removing superior temporal cortical motion areas in the macaque monkey. 1. Motion discrimination using simple dots. *Eur. J. Neurosci.* **4,** 1219–1227.

Cowey, A. & Marcar, V.L. (1992b): The effect of removing superior temporal cortical motion areas in the macaque monkey. 2. Motion discrimination using random dot displays. *Eur. J. Neurosci.* **4,** 1228–1238.

Delis, D.C., Robertson, L.C. & Efron, R. (1986): Hemispheric specialization of memory for visual hierarchical stimuli. *Neuropsychologia* **24,** 205–214.

Desimone, R., Albright, T. & Gross, C. (1984): Stimulus selective properties of inferior temporal neurons in the macaque. *J. Neurosci.* **4,** 2051–2062.

Driver, J. & Mattingley, J.B. (1995): Selective attention in humans: normality and pathology. *Curr. Opinion Neurobiol.* **5,** 191–197.

Egly, R., Driver, J. & Rafal, R.D. (1994a): Shifting visual attention between objects and locations: evidence from normal and parietal lesion subjects. *J. Exp. Psychol.* **123,** 161–177.

Egly, R., Rafal, R., Driver, J. & Starrveveld, Y. (1994b): Covert orienting in the split brain reveals hemispheric specialization for object-based attention. *Psychol. Sci.* **5,** 380–383.

Gainotti, G., Messerli, P. & Tissot, R. (1972): Drawing disability and left and right unilateral retrorolandic brain lesions. *Encéphale* **61,** 245–264.

Goodale, M.A. & Milner, A.D. (1992): Separate visual pathways for perception and action. *Trends Neurosci.* **15,** 20–25.

Haxby, J.V., Grady, C.L., Horwitz, B., Ungerleider, L.G., Mishkin, M., Carson, R.E., Herscovitch, P., Schapiro, M.B. & Rapoport, S.I. (1991): Dissociation of object and spatial visual processing pathways in human extrastriate cortex. *Proc. Nat. Acad. Sci. USA* **88,** 1621–1625.

Haxby, J.V., Horwitz, B., Ungerleider, L.G., Maisog, J.M., Pietrini, P. & Grady, C.L. (1994): The functional organization of human extrastriate cortex: a PET-rCBF study of selective attention to faces and locations. *J. Neurosci.* **14,** 6336–6353.

Heilman, K.M. & Valenstein, E. (1993): *Clinical neuropsychology.* New York, NY: Oxford University Press.

Heilman, K.M. & Van Den Abell, T. (1980): Right hemisphere dominance for attention: the mechanism underlying hemispheric asymmetries of inattention (neglect). *Neurology* **30,** 327–330.

Hess, R.H., Baker Jr., C.L. & Zihl, J. (1989): The 'motion-blind' patient: low-level spatial and temporal filters. *J. Neurosci.* **9,** 1628–1640.

Hillyard, S.A. & Anllo-Vento, L. (1998): Event-related brain potentials in the study of visual selective attention. *Proc. Nat. Acad. Sci. USA* **95 (3),** 781–787.

Hughes, H.C., Fendrich, R. & Reuter-Lorenz, P.A. (1990): Global versus local processing in the absence of low spatial frequencies. *J. Cognitive Neurosci.* **2,** 272–282.

Ivry, R.B. & Robertson, L.C. (1998): *The two sides of perception.* Cambridge, MA: MIT Press.

Jonides, J., Smith, E.E., Koeppe, R.A., Awh, E., Minoshima, S. & Mintun, M.A. (1993): Spatial working memory in humans as revealed by PET. *Nature* **363,** 623–625.

Kanwisher, N. & Driver, J. (1992): Objects, attributes, and visual attention: which, what, and where. *Curr. Dir. Psychol. Sci.* **1,** 26–31.

Kitterle, F.L. & Selig, L.M. (1991): Visual field effects in the discrimination of sine wave gratings. *Perception Psychophysics* **50,** 15–18.

Koffka, K.A. (1935): *Principles of Gestalt psychology.* New York: Harcourt, Brace & World.

Lamb, M.R., Robertson, L.C., Knight, R.T. (1989): Attention and interference in the processing of global and local information: effects of unilateral temporal-parietal junction lesions. *Neuropsychologia* **27,** 471–483.

Lamb, M.R., Robertson, L.C. & Knight, R.T. (1990): Component mechanisms underlying the processing of hierarchically organized patterns: inferences from patients with unilateral cortical lesions. *J. Exp. Psychol.: Learning, Memory, and Cognition,* **16,** 471–483.

Malach, R., Reppas, J.B., Kwong, K.K., Jiang, H., Kennedy, W.A., Ledden, P.J., Brady, T.J., Rosen, B.R. & Tootell, R.B. (1995): Object-related activity revealed by functional magnetic resonance imaging in human occipital cortex. *Proc. Nat. Acad. Sci. USA* **92**, 8135–8139.

Martin, M. (1979): Hemispheric specialization for local and global processing. *Neuropsychologia* **17**, 33–40.

Martinez, A., Anllo-Vento, L. & Hillyard, S.A. (1997a): Brain electrical activity during selective attention to spatial frequency. *Society for Neuroscience Abstracts*.

Martinez, A., Moses, P., Frank, L., Buxton, R., Wong, E. & Stiles, J. (1997b): Hemispheric asymmetries in global and local processing: evidence from fMRI. *Neuroreport* **8**, 1685–1689.

McFie, J., Piercy, M.F. & Zangwill, O.L. (1950): Visualspatial agnosia associated with lesions of the right cerebral hemisphere. *Brain* **73**, 167–190.

Merigan, W.H. & Maunsell, J. (1993): How parallel are the primate visual pathways? *Ann. Rev. Neurosci.* **16**, 369–402.

Mesulam, M.M. (1981): A cortical network for directed attention and unilateral neglect. *Ann. Neurol.* **10**, 309–25.

Mishkin, M., Ungerleider, L.G. & Macko, K.A. (1983): Object vision and spatial vision: two cortical pathways. *Trends Neurosci.* **6**, 414–417.

Newsome, W.T. & Pare, E.B. (1988): A selective impairment of motions perception following lesions of the middle temporal visual area (MT). *J. Neurosci.* **8**, 2201–2211. Perception and action. *Trends Neurosci.* **15**, 20–25.

Posner, M.I. (1980): Orienting of attention. *Quart. J. Exp. Psychol.* **32**, 3–25.

Posner, M.I. & Petersen, S.E. (1990): The attention system of the human brain. *Ann. Rev. Neurosci.* **13**, 25–42.

Posner, M.I., Walker, J.A., Friedrich, F.J. & Rafal, R.D. (1984): Effects of parietal injury on covert orienting of attention. *J. Neurosci.* **4**, 1863–1874.

Rafal, R.D. (1994): Neglect. *Curr. Opinion Neurobiol.* **4**, 231–236.

Rafal, R.D. & Robertson, L. (1995): In: *The neurology of visual attention*, ed. M.S. Gazzaniga. Cambridge, MA: MIT Press.

Robertson, L.C. (1986): *From gestalt to neo-gestalt*. Hillsdale, NJ: Erlbaum.

Robertson, L.C. (1992): Perceptual organization and attentional search in cognitive deficits. In: *Cognitive neuropsychology in clinical practice*, ed. D.I. Margolin. New York: Oxford University Press.

Robertson, L.C. & Lamb, M.R. (1991): Neuropsychological contributions to theories of part/whole organization. *Cognitive Psychol.* **23**, 299–330.

Robertson, L.C., Lamb, M.R. & Knight, R.T. (1988): Effects of lesions of temporal-parietal junction on perceptual and attentional processing in humans. *J. Neurosci.* **8**, 3757–3769.

Robertson, L.C., Lamb, M.R. & Zaidel, E. (1993): Interhemispheric relations in processing hierarchical patterns: evidence from normal and commissurotomized subjects. *Neuropsychology* **7**, 325–342.

Schenk, T. & Zihl, J. (1997): Visual motion perception after brain damage. I. Deficits in global motion perception. *Neuropsychologia* **35**, 1289–1297.

Sergent, J. (1982): The cerebral balance of power: confrontation or cooperation? *J. Exp. Psychol. Hum. Perception Performance* **8**, 253–272.

Shipp, S., de Jong, B.M., Zihl, J., Frackowiak, R. & Zeki, S. (1994): The brain activity related to residual motion vision in a patient with bilateral lesions of V5. *Brain* **117**, 1023–1038.

Shulman, G.L., Sullivan, M.A., Gish, K. & Sakoda, W.J. (1986): The role of spatial frequency channels in the perception of local and global structure. *Perception* **15**, 259–273.

Smith, E.E., Jonides, J. & Koeppe, R.A. (1996): Dissociating verbal and spatial working memory using PET. *Cerebral Cortex* **6**, 11–20.

Smith, E.E., Jonides, J., Koeppe, R.A., Awh, E., Schumacher, E.H. & Minoshima, S. (1995): Spatial versus object working memory: PET investigations. *J. Cognitive Neurosci.* **7,** 337–356.

Tanaka, K., Saito, H., Fukuda, Y. & Moriya, M. (1991): Coding visual images of objects in the inferotemporal cortex of the macaque monkey. *J. Neurophysiol.* **66,** 170–189.

Tipper, S.P. & Behrmann, M. (1996): Object-centered not scene-based visual neglect. *J. Exp. Psychol. Hum. Perception Performance* **22,** 1261–1278.

Tootell, R., Reppas, J.B., Kwong, K.K., Malach, R., Born, R.T., Brady, T.J., Rosen, B.R. & Belliveau, J.W. (1995): Functional analysis of human MT and related visual cortical areas using magnetic resonance imaging. *J. Neurosci.* **15,** 3215–3230.

Treisman, A.M. & Gelade, G. (1980): A feature-integration theory of attention. *Cognitive Psychol.* **12,** 97–136.

Vallar, G. (1993): The anatomical basis of spatial hemineglect in humans. In: *Unilateral neglect: clinical and experimental studies*, Brain damage, behaviour & cognition series, eds. I.H. Robertson & J.C. Marshall, pp. 27–59. Hove, England: Lawrence Erlbaum.

Watson, J., Myers, R., Frackowiak, R., Hajnal, J.V., Woods, R.P., Mazziotta, J.C., Shipp, S. & Zeki, S. (1993): Area V5 of the human brain: evidence from a combined study using positron emission tomography and magnetic resonance imaging. *Cerebral Cortex* **3,** 79–94.

Zeki, S.M. (1978): Functional specialization in the visual cortex of the rhesus monkey. *Nature* **274,** 423–428.

Zeki, S., Watson, J., Lueck, C.J., Friston, K.J., Kennard, C. & Frackowiak, R. (1991): A direct demonstration of functional specialization in human visual cortex. *J. Neurosci.* **11,** 641–649.

Zihl, J., Cramon, D.V. & Mai, N. (1983): Selective disturbance of movement vision after bilateral brain damage. *Brain* **106,** 313–340.

Zihl, J., Cramon, D.V., Mai, N. & Schmid, C.H. (1991): Disturbance of movement vision after bilateral posterior brain damage. *Brain* **114,** 2235–2252.

Chapter 9

Contribution of frontal lobe lesions to cognitive deficit after closed head injury in children

Harvey S. Levin[*] and Sandra B. Chapman[†]

[*]Department of Physical Medicine and Rehabilitation, Baylor College of Medicine, One Baylor Plaza, Houston, Texas 77030, USA; [†]Callier Center for Communication Disorders, University of Texas at Dallas, 1966 Inwood, Dallas, Texas 75235, USA

Summary

In view of the ongoing investigations of cognitive development following head injury in children, caution is advised in extrapolating from this work. However, it is clear from our MRI findings that the prefrontal region is a frequent site of focal lesions after severe head injury in children. Although the overall severity of impaired consciousness contributes to the cognitive sequelae, there is also evidence that focal prefrontal lesions contribute to persistent impairment. An unresolved issue is the relative modularity of subregions of the prefrontal area in children and whether there are differential rates of functional commitment and effects of injury. Specifically, do parallels exist between the dorsolateral-orbitofrontal lesion dissociation in infant monkeys and the sequelae of discrete lesions in these subregions in young children? Is there any evidence for apparent sparing of function after selective prefrontal lesions in young children as compared to older children and adolescents? Our ongoing, longitudinal project has heretofore found no support for initial sparing of function or delayed onset of deficit as children with prefrontal lesions sustained at a young age approach adolescence. However, we are in the process of collecting longitudinal data which will address this issue. Finally, the pattern of executive function deficits in head injured children has implications for devising cognitive interventions to enhance their rehabilitation and special education.

Development of the human prefrontal cortex has been elucidated in neuroanatomic studies which have shown that the density of synaptic contacts peaks by age 11 years (Huttenlocher, 1979). Consistent with the developmental changes in synaptogenesis, positron emission tomography has indicated that the glucose metabolic rate in frontal cortex increases with age, reaching a peak by age 9 years (Chugani *et al.*, 1987). The developmental trajectory of neuroanatomic and metabolic changes is paralleled by major gains and qualitative changes in cognition in children from 6 to 12 years (Case, 1992; Passler *et al.*, 1985). Roberts & Pennington (1996) discuss the possibility that prefrontal maturation results in increased computational or working memory capacity to generate and execute responses and greater inhibitory ability to suppress incorrect prepotent responses. An alternative view is that computational space remains constant, but developmental changes allow the child to reallocate processing resources to cognitive operations which involve online processing of information because basic operations (e.g. reading) become more automatic. However, the relationship between maturational changes of the prefrontal region and cognitive development is poorly understood.

Ablation and reversible lesion experiments (Goldman, 1974; Goldman & Alexander, 1977) in nonhuman primates have shown that subregions of the prefrontal lobes differ in their rate of functional maturation. In 1974 Goldman compared the effects of lesioning the orbitofrontal vs. dorsolateral regions of the frontal lobes on delayed response performance in infant monkeys. This task involved selecting the rewarded side of a two-choice display after observing the examiner bait one of the food cups followed by a delay. In contrast to the initial sparing of function after lesioning the dorsolateral area of the prefrontal region, Goldman found that an orbitofrontal lesion in infant monkeys produced an impairment on the delayed response task which was comparable to that observed after similar lesions in adult monkeys. Follow-up testing at age two years revealed that a delayed response deficit emerged in the monkeys who had dorsolateral lesions as infants. Goldman inferred that the orbitofrontal region was functionally committed during infancy, whereas the dorsolateral region matured later.

Confirmatory observations concerning the heterogeneity of functional maturation of subregions of the frontal lobes in humans are limited, particularly in view of the rarity of discrete lesions confined to one of these areas in children. Although studies of children sustaining discrete prefrontal lesions are sparse, there is minimal evidence for apparent sparing of function analogous to Goldman's observations in infant monkeys subjected to dorsolateral lesions. On the contrary, case reports have suggested that early bifrontal lesions can interfere with cognitive growth, particularly in learning to appreciate the perspective of others and in both moral and social development (Price *et al.*, 1990; Williams & Mateer, 1992). However, developmental studies have raised the possibility that various cognitive capacities subserved by the prefrontal region are heterogeneous in respect of their rate of functional maturation. Using a task analogous to the delayed response, Diamond & Goldman-Rakic (1989) found that human infants between 6 and 12 months began to reach for a location where an object was previously hidden. This finding, which brought into question the view that the prefrontal region becomes functionally mature late in childhood (e.g. at about 10 years), has been interpreted as evidence for the heterogeneous developmental trajectories of the diverse functions subserved by the prefrontal region.

Executive functions and the prefrontal region

The term 'executive function' (EF) refers to the distinct, but related cognitive abilities which depend primarily on a network or system comprised by the prefrontal area and its major connections. Although this definition (or its variants) is widely accepted, there is no consensus concerning the specific cognitive abilities which comprise EFs. To build consensus on this aspect of cognitive development, the National Institute of Child Health and Development in the United States sponsored a workshop in 1994 which focused on EFs in children. The workshop proceedings reflected the diversity of EFs and our rudimentary understanding of interrelationships. It was also clear that there is variation in the purported relationship of development to the maturation of various subregions of the prefrontal region. While acknowledging these limitations, the workshop participants reached consensus on the following EFs:

Flexibility in problem solving

This refers to the capacity for shifting response strategy according to changes in the environment. This ability has been traditionally tested by changing the rewarded dimension (e.g. from colour to shape) and assessing the individual's ability to shift strategy on the Wisconsin Card Sorting Test (Grant & Berg, 1948). From the perspective of Roberts & Pennington (1996) which stresses growth of inhibitory capacity for suppressing inappropriate responses, the tendency to respond according to the previously correct dimension decreases with age as the child becomes more capable of inhibiting prepotent responses. According to this view, flexibility in problem solving is intrinsically related to inhibitory capacity. Tasks which involve generation of exemplars of categories, words beginning with a specific letter (Benton, 1968), or unique designs (Jones-Gotman & Milner, 1977), are also viewed as measures of flexibility in problem solving.

Temporal organization of behaviour

Delayed response experiments in nonhuman primates have documented that prefrontal neurons become active during the delay interval (Fuster, 1989). As noted above, the capacity for organizing behaviour over time while maintaining a stimulus in 'working memory' emerges during the second half of the first year in human infants. The capacity to maintain an internal representation of a stimulus over time is intrinsic to this EF.

Planning

This EF refers to the capacity for setting goals and maintaining an action sequence in working memory. Cognitive neuropsychologists have also characterized the ability to break a complex into subsidiary goals as a feature of planning. Shallice (1982) designed the Tower of London to assess planning. The subject's task is to rearrange the beads on three rods to match a model using as few moves as possible. Performance on problems of varying complexity, which differ in the number of moves necessary for solution, is measured by the percentage of problems solved on the first trial and within the maximum number of trials (e.g. a limit of three trials per problem is used in our laboratory). Shallice (1982) reported that this task was specifically impaired in adults with anterior brain lesions, a finding which was confirmed by Owen et al. (1990). Although the distinction between planning and the temporal organization of behaviour is ambiguous, the former tends to emphasize formulating a sequence of responses whereas the latter stresses maintaining an internal representation over a delay.

Resource allocation

This EF refers to the computational capacity for online manipulation or transformation of information such as performing concurrent tasks which involve divided attention. The ability to redistribute attention to one or the other task (e.g. a child taking notes while listening to the teacher's lecture) is assessed in studies of divided attention which test reaction time while subjects perform a target detection task or a verbal task such as proofreading to find errors.

Inhibition

In proposing inhibition as an EF, the workshop participants referred to the capacity for switching from initiation to termination of a response at the appropriate time. This active view of inhibition also implies that the subject inhibits less appropriate responses while selecting the appropriate response. Other features include resistance to interference by distracters or conflicting response tendencies (e.g. performing the Stroop Test which involves suppressing the prepotent response of reading words instead of naming the colour of print as instructed by the examiner (Perret, 1974). Other measures of inhibition include Go–No Go and continuous performance tasks which involve responding rapidly to a target and withholding response to distracters.

Self regulation

This EF refers to the capacity for self-monitoring, including cognitive perfomance such as utilizing strategies to enhance memory or study skills and the capacity to monitor one's behaviour in relation to external constraints or according to an internal representation which guides behaviour. Other features of this EF include Luria's emphasis on self-regulation by verbal mediation and the use of self-evaluation to modulate emotional reactions. Features of self monitoring include its 'on-line' status and engagement of prospective memory rather than episodic memory and past behaviour.

Working memory

Pennington (1994) has incorporated several of the aforementioned EFs in his definition of working memory 'as a capacity limited system which maintains internal representations on-line while inhibiting other information. Working memory is transient, context dependent, and prospective involving planning, monitoring, and organizing memory' (p. 248).

Development of executive functions in children

In preparation for investigating the sequelae of prefrontal lesions, Levin et al. (1991) studied normal children who comprised the age groups 7–8 years, 9–12 years, and adolescents 13–15 years. The tasks administered included the Wisconsin Card Sorting Test, word and design fluency, Twenty Questions (Denney & Denney, 1973), Go–No Go (Drewe, 1975), Tower of London (Shallice, 1982), and the California Verbal Learning Test (Delis et al., 1986). The results depicted a developmental trend on these measures of EF. Figure 1 indicates that flexibility in problem solving increased with age as reflected by the percentage of categories (the maximum number was six), the increased percentage of conceptual level responses (i.e. three consecutively correct sorts), and the decreased percentage of preservative errors. Statistical analysis indicated that most of the age-related change occurred between the 7–8 years olds and the older groups.

Similar developmental trends of enhanced problem solving skills were confirmed on the Twenty Questions and fluency tasks. Figure 2 shows that the percentage of constraint responses (i.e. excluding several exemplars of a conceptual category by asking a question such as 'Is it a living thing?') increased with age. In contrast, the percentage of questions which referred to only a single item (i.e. hypothesis-seeking questions) declined in the older children. Planning ability, as measured by the Tower of London, also increased particularly for problems of intermediate complexity.

Utilizing the Go–No Go task, Levin et al. (1991) found that the number of false alarm errors (i.e. responding to the negative signal) and misses (failing to respond to a target) decreased with age (Fig. 3). This pattern of changes is consistent with the view that inhibitory control increases with age. The greatest developmental shift appears to occur from 7–8 to 9–12 years.

Taken together, this cross-sectional study indicates impressive gains in flexibility of problem solving, planning and inhibition by age 12 years. A more gradual developmental trend was

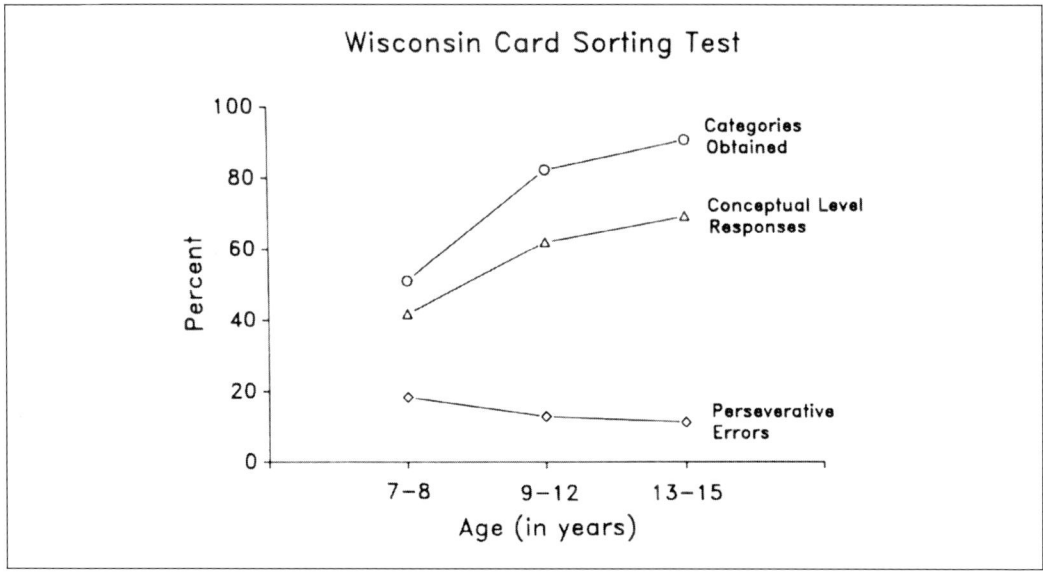

Fig. 1. Performance on the WCST plotted against age group in normal children. Number of categories obtained (expressed as a percentage of total categories), percentage of conceptual level responses, and percentage of perseverative errors are shown. Reproduced from Levin et al. (1991).

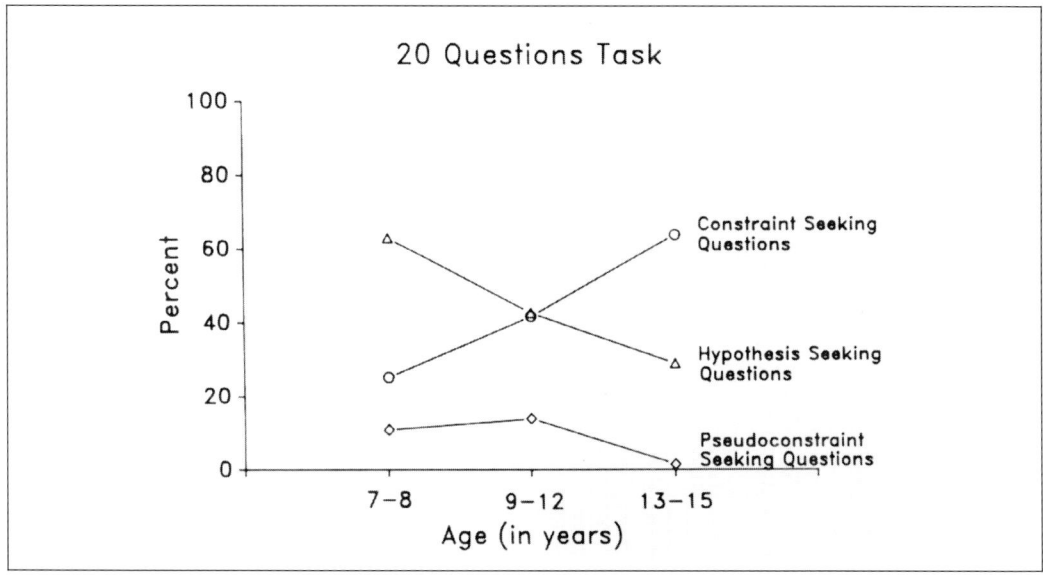

Fig. 2. The percentage of constraint-seeking questions, hypothesis-seeking questions, and pseudoconstraint seeking questions plotted against age of normal children. Reproduced from Levin et al. (1991).

found for utilizing semantic information in formulating questions as reflected by the major gains in adolescents relative to the younger groups. Based on these findings, Levin et al. (1991) inferred that prefrontal injury occurring in children older than 8 years is more likely to produce unequivocal impairments of concept formation, cognitive flexibility and inhibitory capacity.

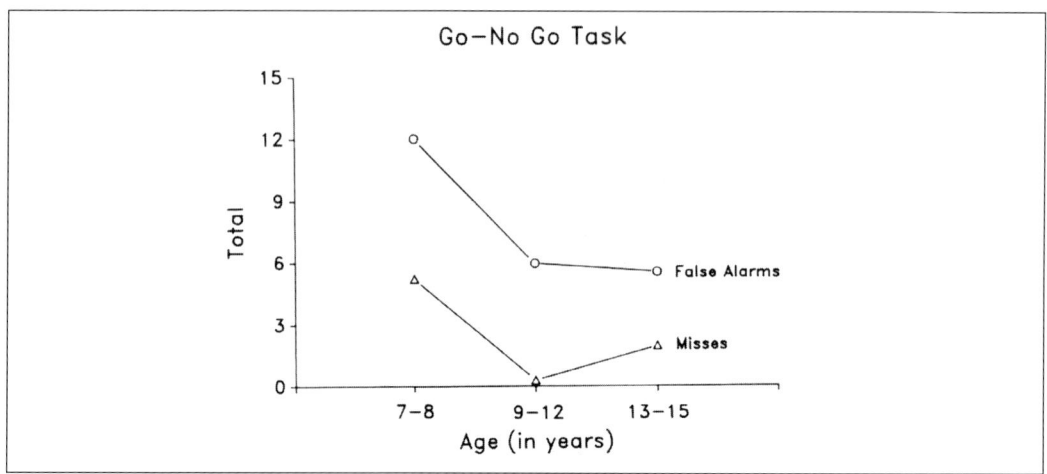

Fig. 3. Total number of false-positive responses ('False Alarms') and number of misses on the Go–No Go Task as a function of age in normal children. Reproduced from Levin et al. (1991).

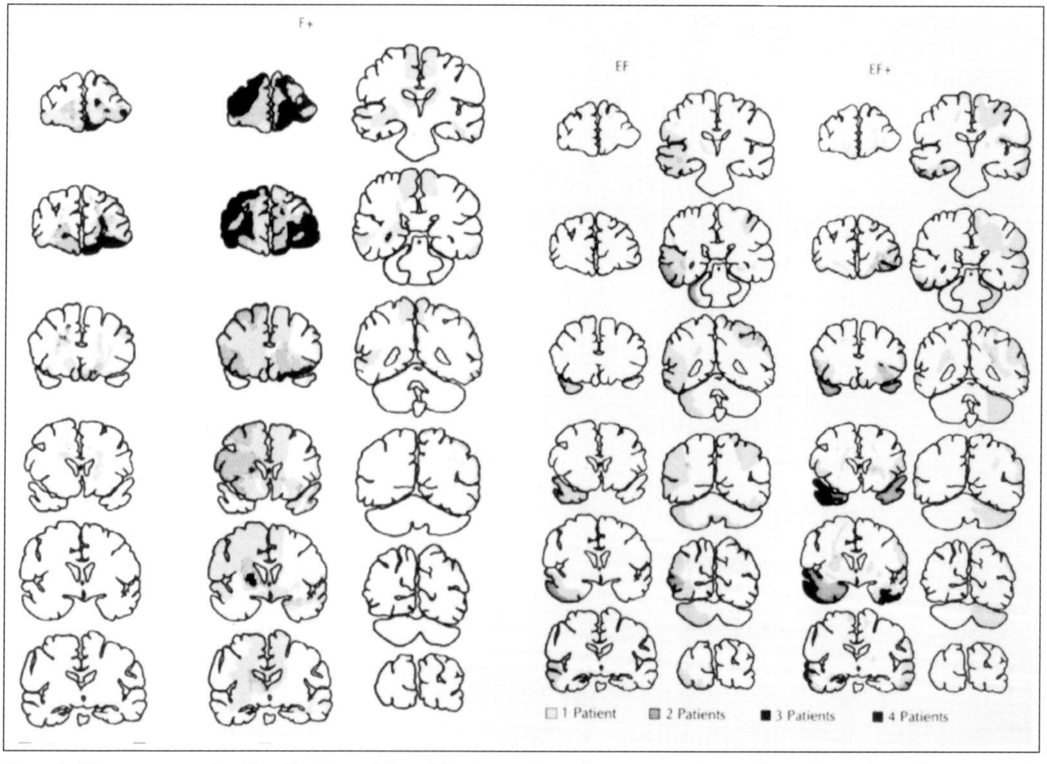

Fig. 4. Neuroanatomic distribution of focal lesions plotted on coronal templates based on the magnetic resonance imaging (MRI) findings of 57 head injured paediatric patients. Left, focal lesions of 20 patients whose areas of abnormal signal were confined to the frontal lobes (F) and the group (F+) whose lesions primarily involved the frontal lobes but extended to extrafrontal regions (n = 11). Right, the areas of abnormal signal for children (n = 15) whose MRI findings were confined to the extrafrontal region (EF), and MRI findings in children (n = 11) with predominantly extrafrontal (EF+) lesions that encroached on the frontal area. Reproduced from Levin et al. (1993).

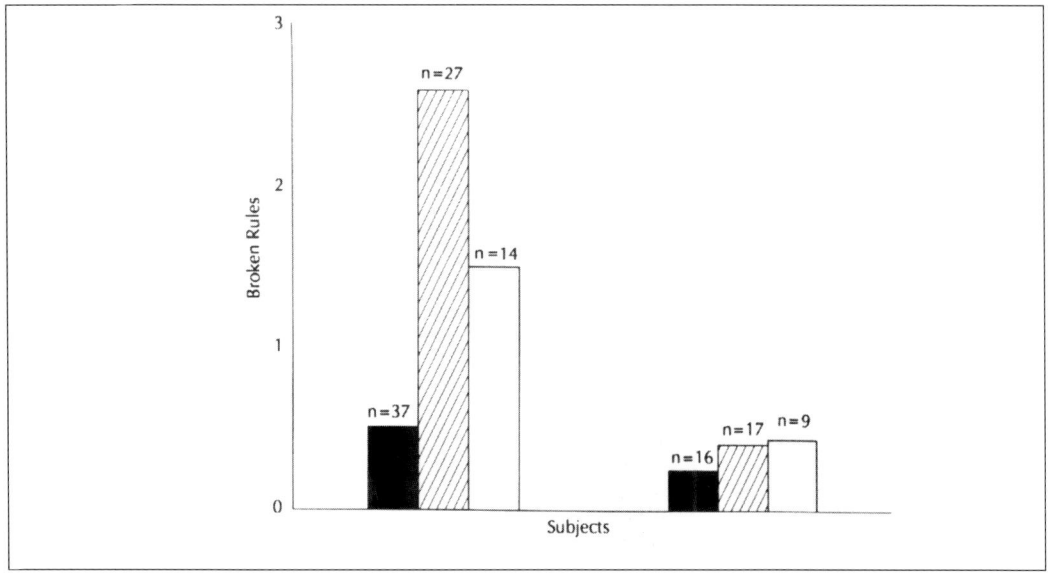

Fig. 5. Number of broken rules incurred while completing the Tower of London task for controls (closed bars), head-injured children with GCS scores of 8 or less (hatched bars), and head-injured children with GCS scores greater than 8 (open bars). Means are shown for 6–10 year-old (left) and 11–16 year-old (right) groups. Reproduced from Levin et al. (1993).

Relationship of prefrontal lesions to cognitive deficits following closed head injury

To characterize the presence and sequelae of persistent focal brain lesions after CHI, Levin *et al.* (1993) completed a cross-sectional study of 76 children and adolescents who had sustained a CHI of varying severity at least 3 months earlier. The patients were divided into groups according to their age at the time of the study (i.e. 6–10, 11–16 years) and their severity of acute impairment of consciousness as measured by the Glasgow Coma Scale (GCS) of Teasdale & Jennett (1974) (i.e. GCS score ≤ 8, ≥ 9). MRI was performed within one week of the cognitive assessment which included the measures used in the developmental study (Levin *et al.*, 1991). Normal children were selected from the same community to serve in comparison groups for the 6–10 and 11–16 year ranges.

The MRI findings disclosed that 75 per cent of the head injured patients had focal areas of abnormal signal which were consistent with a brain lesion, including gliosis (70 per cent of the lesions), encephalomalacia (13 per cent of the lesions), hemosiderin deposit (4 per cent of the lesions), hygroma (4 per cent), and atrophy (4 per cent). Figure 4 displays the neuronatomic distribution of lesions in the head injured patients, reflecting a rostrocaudal gradient. Forty per cent of the head injured patients had a lesion either confined to or primarily in the prefrontal region, whereas only 15 per cent of the sample had an extrafrontal lesion which did not encroach on the prefrontal region.

All of the cognitive tests were sensitive to the severity of CHI and the age of the patients and controls. In addition to the overall effects of injury severity and age, there was some evidence for increased vulnerability to injury effects in young children on the Tower of London (Fig. 5). Head injured children in the 6–10 years age range incurred far more broken rules (e.g. picking up more than one bead at a time) than head injured adolescents and normal controls. This

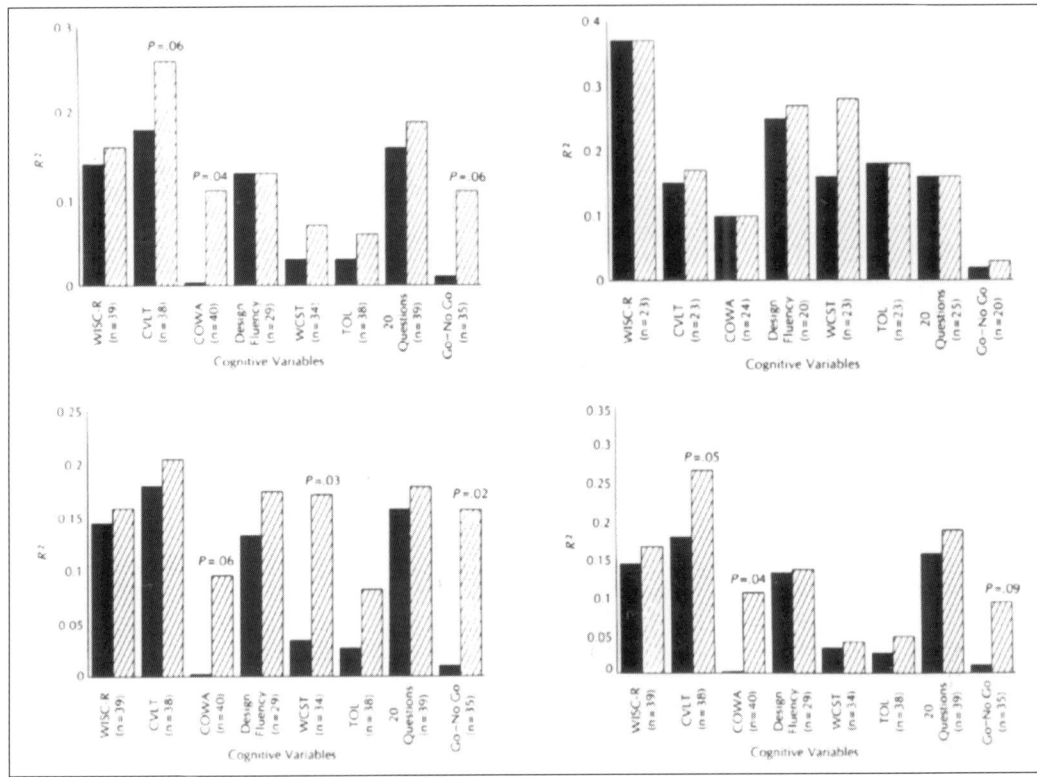

Fig. 6. Summary of the results of hierarchical multiple regression that evaluated the contributions of frontal (top left) and extrafrontal (top right) lesions to making incremental the variance in cognitive test scores explained by the lowest postresuscitation GCS score. The regressions were repeated to evaluate specifically the contributions of left frontal (bottom left) and right frontal (bottom right) lesions. Closed bars indicate R^2; hatched bars indicate incremental R^2.
Wisc-R: Wechsler Intelligence Scale for Children-Revised; CVLT: California Verbal Learning Test; COWA: Controlled Oral Word Association; WCST: Wisconsin Card Sorting Test; TOL: Tower of London. Reproduced from Levin et al. (1993).

finding was particularly salient because the examiner reminded the child each time a rule was broken.

To analyse the relationship of focal brain lesions to cognitive function, Levin *et al.* (1993) used multiple regression in which the severity of injury (i.e. GCS score) and the child's age were first entered into the regression equation and the volume of lesion in a designated region was entered to determine its incremental contribution to cognitive test performance as indexed by the R2 on the y-axis (Fig. 6). The addition of left frontal lesions to the regression equation enhanced prediction of Wisconsin Card Sorting and Go–No Go performance while the incremental prediction of controlled oral word association (COWA) (word fluency) was nearly significant. A similar analysis of right frontal lesions produced significant incremental effects for semantic clustering on the California Verbal Learning Test and word association while enhanced prediction of Go–No Go performance approached significance. In contrast, Fig. 6 shows that extrafrontal lesion volume was not predictive of any cognitive measure. In summary, our findings indicate that measures of EF in children are sensitive to the severity of CHI and to

Chapter 9 Contribution of frontal lobe lesions to cognitive deficit after closed head injury in children

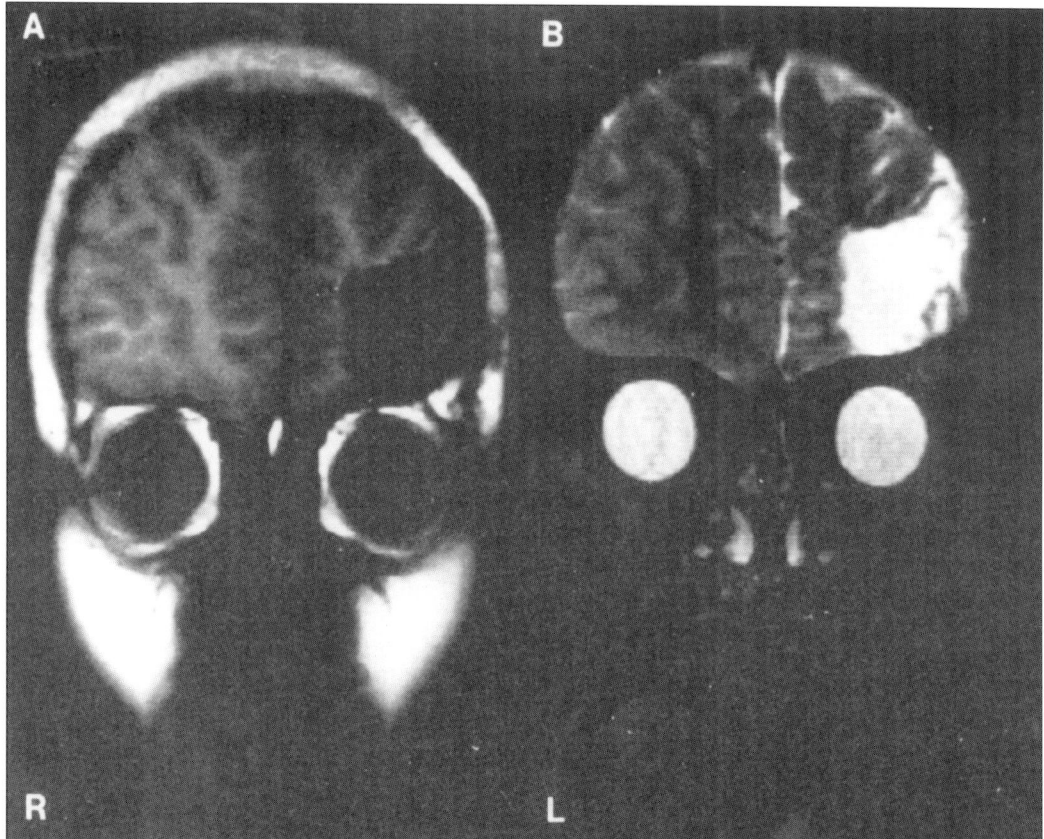

Fig. 7. T1- and T2-weighted (repetition time 300/20 and 3000/120 ms) coronal MRI scans performed two years after patient 1 sustained a severe closed head injury (age 7 years 6 months). The scans disclosed a large area of post-traumatic encephalomalacia measuring approximately 2.8 x 2.8 x 2.5 cm (craniocaudal, transverse, anteroposterior) within the anteroinferior aspect of the left frontal lobe, involving the orbitofrontal inferior and middle frontal gyri and the adjacent underlying frontal white matter. Reproduced from Levin et al. (1993).

the volume of prefrontal lesions. Longitudinal investigation is in progress to assess whether the degree of deficit increases with age.

The findings obtained through statistical analysis of group data can be appreciated through a summary of an individual patient.

Case report

A 5 year 4 month old right-handed boy sustained a severe CHI when he was struck by a car. The GCS score was 6 on hospital admission. Serial CT scans during the initial hospitalization revealed multiple left frontotemporal contusions. An MRI scan at two years postinjury (Fig. 7) showed left frontal traumatic encephalomalacia involving the inferior and middle frontal gyri and the frontal white matter. Behavioural sequelae included attention disturbance, overtalkativeness, mild disinhibition, memory problems, and mild difficulty with language comprehension. Although he returned to regular second grade classes and obtained average scores on the

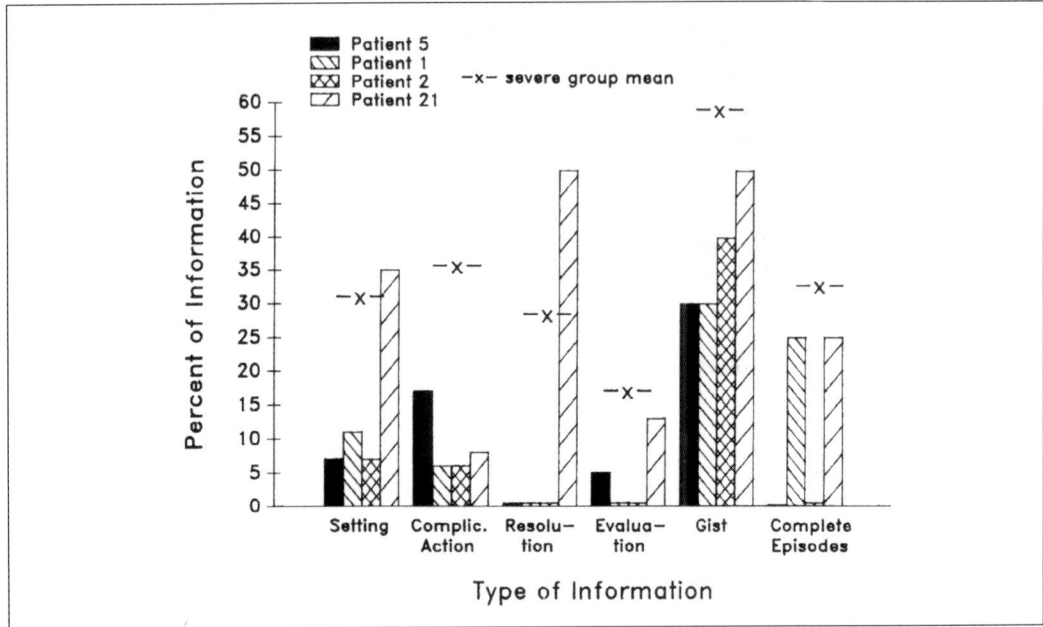

Fig. 8. Comparison of four subjects with frontal lobe damage with the mean for the severely injured closed head injury group (indicated by 'x') on measures of information structure in discourse. Reproduced from Chapman et al. (1992).

WISC-R (Verbal IQ, 105, Performance IQ, 92) at two years following injury, his scores on specific cognitive tests were highly variable. In contrast to performance on the Wisconsin Card Sorting Test and Tower of London which was within the normal range, he failed to use constraint-seeking questions on the Twenty Questions Test. Verbal fluency was deficient and he underutilized semantic clustering to organize recall. He was unable to reach criterion within 40 trials on the Go–No Go test.

These findings reflect the intraindividual variability of cognitive functioning after severe injury to the left prefrontal region in a child. This case also illustrates the inadequacy of limiting follow-up assessment to a standard measure of intellectual ability.

Narrative discourse after closed head injury

Previous studies have disclosed that discourse processing deficits are common in adults following CHI, including patients whose language appears to be recovered when tested on measures at a single word level such as naming (Ehrlich, 1988). The relationship of prefrontal lesions to discourse processing deficits has also been reported (Alexander et al., 1989), particularly in regard to drawing inferences, and appreciating the gist or essential information. Dennis & Barnes (1990) reported that discourse representation is impaired following CHI in children, an observation which raised a question concerning the features which are most vulnerable. The organizational structure (i.e. chronology of events and semantic content) in narrative discourse is a feature which might be predisposed to impairment following CHI. To elucidate the nature of narrative discourse deficits after CHI in paediatric CHI, Chapman et al. (1992) studied various domains of narrative discourse in 20 children and adolescents who had sustained a CHI and had an MRI scan to characterize focal brain lesions. Chapman et al. analysed three domains of the children's narrative discourse (i.e. retelling stories immediately after they were presented by the examiner), including language structure (e.g. total number of words, clauses); information structure (i.e. number of propositions or information units, global story content or gist information, story organization, setting, sequence of events, and resolution); and flow of information (i.e. to assess disruptions in the flow of information). Analysis of the transcribed stories disclosed that in comparison with the discourse of a normal control group, children who had sustained severe CHI exhibited a reduction in the amount of language (domain I), but not in the complexity of language. The most dramatic differences were found in the information content and the organization. For examples, their stories were marked by reductions in both gist and episodic information (domain II). Utilizing an analysis of covariance, Chapman *et al.* were able to show that the discourse processing deficits could not be explained by impairment in lexical retrieval or immediate recall. This disruption of story content and structure was interpreted by Chapman and co-workers as consistent with clinical observations that the discourse of patients following severe CHI is often disorganized.

To explore the relationship between focal brain lesions and discourse processing, Chapman *et al.* identified four children whose MRI revealed focal areas of abnormal signal situated in the prefrontal region (including two patients with left frontal lesions, a child with right superior frontal gyrus and orbital frontal lesions, and a case with bifrontal lesions). Figure 8 plots the percentage of information included in the narratives of these children and the mean scores for all nine children who had sustained a severe CHI irrespective of their MRI findings. The narratives of all four children with frontal lesions were deficient in various types of information pertaining to story structure (e.g. setting) and macrostructure (i.e. gist) which differed both across the individual patients and within a single subject. Figure 8 indicates that all four children included less gist information than the mean level for the severe CHI group and that only one of the four patients was able to explain the resolution of the stories to a level comparable to severely injured patients without prefrontal lesions. In contrast to the findings for the language and information structures, the flow of information in the narratives of the four patients with frontal lesions was comparable to that of the severe CHI group. Whether or not the deficits in discourse organization are associated with impairments in EFs (e.g. planning, temporary organization of behaviour, or inhibition) remains to be determined.

Acknowledgements: This research was funded in part by NIH grant NS-21889. The authors wish to thank Angela D. Williams for word processing and editorial assistance.

References

Alexander, M.P., Benson, D.F. & Stuss, D.T. (1989): Frontal lobes and language. *Brain Lang.* **37**, 656–691.

Benton, A.L. (1968): Differential behavioral effects in frontal lobe disease. *Neuropsychologia* **6**, 53–60.

Case, R. (1992): The role of the frontal lobes in the regulation of cognitive development. *Brain Cognition* **20**, 51–73.

Chapman, S.B., Culhane, K.A., Levin, H.S., Harward, H., Mendelsohn, D., Ewing-Cobbs, L., Fletcher, J.M. & Bruce, D. (1992): Narrative discourse after closed head injury in children and adolescents. *Brain Lang.* **43**, 42–65.

Chugani, H.T., Phelps, M.E. & Mazziotta, J.C. (1987): Positron emission tomography study of human brain functional development. *Ann. Neurol.* **22**, 487–497.

Delis, D.C., Kramer, J.H., Kaplan, E. & Ober, B.A. (1986): *The California Verbal Learning Test* – Research Edition. New York: Psychological Corp.

Denney, D.R. & Denney, N.W. (1973): The use of classification for problem-solving: a comparison of middle and old age. *Dev. Psychol.* **9**, 275–278.

Dennis, M. & Barnes, M.A. (1990): Knowing the meaning, getting the point, bridging the gap, and carrying the message: aspects of discourse following closed head injury in childhood and adolescence. *Brain Lang.* **39**, 428–446.

Diamond, A. & Goldman-Rakic, P.S. (1989): Comparison of human infants and rhesus monkeys on Piaget's A-not-B task: evidence for dependence on dorsolateral prefrontal cortex. *Exp. Brain Res.* **74**, 24–40.

Drewe, E.A. (1975): Go-no go learning after frontal lobe lesions in humans. *Cortex* **11**, 8–16.

Ehrlich, J.S. (1988): Selective characteristics of narrative discourse in head-injured and normal adults. *J. Comm. Disorders* **21**, 1–9.

Fuster, J.M. (1989): *The prefrontal cortex. Anatomy, physiology and neuropsychology of the frontal lobe*, 2nd edn. New York: Raven Press.

Goldman, P.S. (1974): Functional recovery after lesions of the nervous systems. 3. Developmental processes in neural plasticity. Recovery of function after CNS lesions in infant monkeys. *Neurosci. Res. Progr. Bull.* **12**, 217–222.

Goldman, P.S. & Alexander, G.E. (1977): Maturation of prefrontal cortex in the monkey revealed by focal reversible cryogenic depression. *Nature* **267**, 613–615.

Grant, D.A. & Berg, E.A. (1948): A behavioral analysis of degree of reinforcement and ease of shifting to a new response in a Weigl type card sorting problem. *J. Exp. Psychol.* **38**, 404–411.

Huttenlocher, P.R. (1979): Synaptic density in human frontal cortex: developmental changes and effects of aging. *Brain Res.* **163**, 195–205.

Jones-Gotman, M. & Milner, B. (1977): Design fluency: the inventions of nonsense drawings after focal cortical lesions. *Neuropsychologia* **15**, 653–674.

Levin, H.S., Culhane, K.A., Hartmann, J., Evankovich, D., Mattson, A.J., Harward, H., Ringholz, G., Ewing-Cobbs, L. & Fletcher, J.M. (1991): Developmental changes in performance on tests of purported frontal lobe functioning. *Dev. Neuropsychol.* **7**, 377–395.

Levin, H.S., Culhane, K.A., Mendelsohn, D., Lilly, M.A., Bruce, D., Fletcher, J.H.M., Chapman, S.B., Harward, H. & Eisenberg, H.M. (1993): Cognition in relation to MRI in head injured children and adolescents. *Arch. Neurol.* **50**, 897–905.

Owen, A.M., Downes, J.J., Sahakian, B.J., Polkey, C.E. & Robbins, T.W. (1990): Planning and spatial working memory following frontal lobe lesions in man. *Neuropsychologia* **28**, 1021–1034.

Passler, M.A., Isaac, W. & Hynd, G.W. (1985): Neuropsychological development of behavior attributed to frontal lobe functioning in children. *Dev. Neuropsychol.* **1**, 349–370.

Pennington, B.F. (1994): The working memory function of the prefrontal cortices: implications for developmental and individual differences in cognition. In: *The development of future oriented processes*, eds. M.M. Haith, J. Benson, R.J. Roberts, Jr. & B.F. Pennington, pp. 243–289. Chicago: University of Chicago Press.

Perret, E. (1974): The left frontal lobe in man and suppression of habitual responses in verbal categorical behavior. *Neuropsychologia* **12**, 232–330.

Price, B.H., Daffner, K.R., Stowe, R.M. & Mesulam, M.M. (1990): The comportmental learning disabilities of early frontal lobe damage. *Brain* **113**, 1383–1393.

Roberts, R.J. & Pennington, B.F. (1996): An interactive framework for examining prefrontal cognitive processes. *Dev. Neuropsychol.* **12**, 105–126.

Shallice, T. (1982): Specific impairments of planning. Philosophical transactions of the Royal Society of London. *Biology* **298**, 199–209.

Teasdale, G. & Jennett B. (1974): Assessment of coma and impaired consciousness: a practical scale. *Lancet* **ii**, 81–84.

Williams, D. & Mateer, C.A. (1992): Developmental impact of frontal lobe injury in middle childhood. *Brain Cognition* **20**, 196–204.

Chapter 10

Agnosias

Francesca Nichelli and Daria Riva

Divisione di Neurologia dello Sriluppo, Istituto Nazionale Neurologico Carlo Besta, Via Celoria 11, 20133 Milan, Italy

Summary

This chapter describes disturbances relating to the recognition of objects (agnosia) and faces (prosopagnosia). The neuropsychological investigation of adult cases still uses the classification of apperceptive and associative agnosia introduced by Lissauer & Freud, whereas more recent cognitive models (Humphreys & Riddoch, 1987; Bruce & Young, 1986) provide a useful explanation of the fine differences encountered in clinical practice. The processes of object and face recognition both require different stages of stimulus analysis, which may be individually impaired without affecting the others. The few published studies concerning children seem to confirm the methods of processing objects and faces described in adults. Nevertheless, there is a need to explore this further by using methods that are more appropriate for childhood population, and which take cases presenting cerebral lesions or malformations into greater account.

Introduction

The first studies of the neuropsychological deficits relating to object recognition were carried out at the end of the 19th century, and their current classification still uses the terminology introduced by Lissauer (1890) and Freud (1891).

Lissauer proposed distinguishing the deficits affecting the ability to discriminate stimuli and perceive consciously from those affecting the ability to interpret what is seen. These two subtypes were respectively defined *apperceptive* and *associative* 'mental blindness'. However, the concept of mental blindness was very generic and based on theoretical data rather than empirical observations; it consisted of a broad group of disturbances, including the ability to distinguish colours and identify differences between new shapes and models, as well as specific disturbances relating to the perception of objects. Lissauer described a patient (Gottlieb L.) who made mistakes in identifying everyday objects. He appeared confused when he tried using cutlery to eat and had difficulty in dressing himself, but was able to copy drawings and showed no signs of any intellectual deficit. According to Lissauer, this was an example of associative blindness. However, the descriptions of apperceptive disturbances were rather vague, being seen more as a prerequisite for the onset of other disturbances than as a specific deficit in itself.

In the year following the publication of Lissauer's article, Freud introduced the term *agnosia*, thus further specifying the concept of mental blindness. He held that agnosic deficits should not be considered simple disturbances in sensorial processing, but as indicators of damage affecting previously learnt knowledge.

These concepts of Lissauer and Freud provide a useful starting point for analysing object recognition disturbances. The discontinuity between what Lissauer called associative and apperceptive disturbances, and what Freud called sensory and gnosic disturbances, makes it possible to distinguish: (1) deficits involving sensory processing (elementary sensory disturbances); (2) deficits concerning the perceptive analysis of stimuli (apperceptive agnosia); and (3) deficits in the analysis of the semantic, functional and structural analysis of stimuli (associative agnosia).

We shall here leave aside elementary sensorial disturbances (cortical blindness, colour discrimination disorders, the perception of movement, depth, etc.) and concentrate on those that are more strictly related to object recognition.

In order to be able to speak of agnosia, a patient's recognition difficulties must be limited to one sensory channel and not be attributable to elementary perception disturbances, eye-movement disorders, attention deficits, aphasic language alterations or intellectual deficit.

Apperceptive agnosia

The greatest difficulty in terms of diagnosis is to determine the limits of the alterations in primary visual functions that are compatible with a picture of agnosia. In order to be able to speak of a selective perceptual deficit, it is necessary to demonstrate the existence of sufficient sensory visual capacities; consequently, visual field, visual acuity, and the discrimination of colours and depth must all be normal.

Patients with apperceptive agnosia fail at object recognition tasks because they are unable to organize sensory data into the structured perceptual units that make it possible to reconstruct their shape and so recognize them. The tests at which they are deficient are those requiring the recognition of objects seen from an untypical angle, the identification of a particular figure mixed with others in an overlapping complex, the matching of identical drawings of different sizes, and the copying of drawings.

The lesion responsible for apperceptive agnosia generally involves the right parietal lobe. Studies have shown that patients with right posterior lesions are capable of performing shape discrimination tests within the limits of normal levels, but are severely impaired when it comes to tests involving unconventional perspectives and incomplete figures (Warrington & Taylor, 1973).

This finding is confirmed by the results obtained in a large number of individual case studies. Humphreys & Riddoch (1984) studied two patients who had severe disturbances in recognizing objects photographed from unusual angles, but whose performances were normal at tests in which they had to decide whether two lines were parallel, or assess the length of lines or the size of circles. Warrington & James (1988) found that, although their patients were capable of identifying a destructured 'X' presented on a confused background, they had great difficulties in identifying individual destructured letters. De Renzi *et al.* (1989) also observed that patients with right posterior lesions preserved the ability to distinguish stimuli. Further confirmation of an intact capacity to identify a stimulus in the presence of a figure identification deficit have been reported in the case of stereopsis evaluation tests (Benton & Hécaen, 1970). Taken together, these results suggest a certain degree of discontinuity between sensory visual processing and the processes involved in object perception.

The first interpretation of apperceptive agnosia was made by Warrington & James (1988), who defined it as a disturbance of the perceptive categorization that makes it possible to provide a structural definition of objects (i.e. their distinctive elements and the spatial relationships between them). This definition is based on Marr's object recognition computational model (Marr, 1980, 1982), and divides the representation of a visual stimulus into three distinct stages.

According to Warrington, all objects must be analysed on the basis of their sensory visual properties. At this first level of processing, there is no functional lateralization and the information is represented retinotopically. The second stage gives rise to a perceptive classification and is lateralized to the right hemisphere. The third stage makes it possible to assign a meaning to what is perceived and therefore to create a semantic classification.

In the second stage (the storage of the structural knowledge of objects), every percept is specified by a substantial number of characteristics and their relative (not absolute) spatial positions. In this way, a group of distinct elements and their reciprocal relationships characterize the structural identity of an object, and it is this that makes the object recognisable despite any changes in form, size or the visual angle from which it is seen (including untypical perspectives, face-on or in profile, or when it needs to be recognized on the basis of an incomplete representation). Warrington's interpretation has the advantage of explaining the deficits shown by patients with apperceptive agnosia when doing those tasks in which an object's distinctive structural characteristics are less evident, such as when they are obscured (the overlapping figures of Poppelreuter and Ghent), destructured (the incomplete figures of Gollin) or distorted (shown from untypical angles).

A model of the functional components involved in object recognition and naming has been proposed by Humphreys & Riddoch (1987), whose model makes use of perception processing modules that may be lesioned individually and independently of each other. These authors do not limit themselves to the classical division between apperceptive and associative agnosia, but also identify other forms on the basis of the processing level of the lesioned stimulus. Perceptive deficit can therefore manifest itself at any level and give rise to three distinct forms of agnosia: shape agnosia, integrative agnosia and transformational agnosia.

In the case of *shape agnosia*, patients are capable of automatically decoding the individual characteristics of the stimulus in a parallel manner, but fail to process the shape as a whole. A deficit at this level can be seen in the patients described by Adler (1950), Efron (1968), and Campion & Latto (1985). The disturbance is manifested by an inability to trace the outlines of a stimulus, match identical stimuli, distinguish forms from their background, and differentiate geometric forms. As a consequence, patients do not recognize objects even when they appear in their canonical position, especially if they are represented in the form of two-dimensional drawings.

In the case of *integrative agnosia*, the impaired stage corresponds to the integration of the individual perceptive characteristics of a form (its outlines, internal details, etc.) into a single unit. One exemplary case has been described by Humphreys & Riddoch (1987): after experiencing a bilateral occipital infarction, the patient retained good visual acuity and discrimination of length but, in everyday life, had difficulty in or took a long time over recognizing objects. He was prosopagnosic, acromatoptic, disoriented in space, and read single words with great difficulty. He could match drawings of the same object looked at from different perspectives and was capable of accurately copying even those he was unable to identify. However, the copying was very slow and laborious, detail after detail, as if he had difficulty in integrating the various elements of a figure into a significant structure. His slowness was also evident when he did tasks involving the identification of overlapping figures or figures presented tachistoscopically during a decision-making test concerning the reality of unreal figures (animals or objects to which a non-existent detail had been added, or in which an important detail had been replaced by something incongruous). In one version, the stimuli were presented to the patient in the form of drawings mixed with others of real objects; in another, they were black silhouettes devoid of any internal details. The patient's performance was deficient with both versions, but his disturbance was much less evident in the case of the silhouettes because, unlike the drawings, this type of stimulus did not require the integration of a large number of details into a single percept. The authors therefore hypothesized that the patient was capable of recognizing the overall shape of the stimulus and the details taken one at a time, but not capable of integrating them.

In the classification of Humphreys & Riddoch (1987), *transformational agnosia* corresponds to what Warrington (1985) understands by apperceptive agnosia: that is, a deficit in perceptive categorization. Patients cannot use the procedures necessary to transform the perceptive structure of the analysed stimulus (variations in perspective, distance, lighting conditions, etc.), and it therefore becomes impossible to compare the perceptive image corresponding to the seen object with the interior knowledge stored in its prototypical form. The abstract representation of a structure arises from a multiplicity of perceptive experiences; it is this that allows it to be recognized under various conditions of distance, lighting, perspective, etc., regardless of the point of view of the observer. It is a representation centred on the object itself. The constitutive element of such a representation (which belongs to Marr's 3-D level) is not the main axis of the shape (as Marr supposed), but its significant details: i.e. the set of visual outlines and spatial relationships that gives an object its individuality. A right (generally parietal) lesion alters this representation and therefore the recognition of the perceptive category of the stimulus unless it is presented in canonical positions.

To be considered such, transformational agnosia must not be associated with a disturbance of internal visual representation (mental images), and so the patient must be able to draw figures from memory.

Associative agnosia

One can speak of associative agnosia when it is possible for patients to analyse and integrate the perceptive structure of the stimulus, and when there are no alterations in its internal representation. A pure deficit of this type is quite rare: in a study involving 415 subjects, Hécaen & Angelergues (1963) found four cases, only one of which was free of other cognitive disturbances. De Renzi & Spinnler (1966) found one case in a study of 122 patients.

The tests that patients with associative agnosia fail to complete successfully are those requiring a knowledge of an object's functional and semantic characteristics. As a consequence, there may be many semantic errors in a visual denomination task, considerable difficulties in a test involving semantic categorization (grouping stimuli belonging to the same category, selecting those figures from a group that have close associative links, etc.), and difficulties relating to semantic attributes that are not present in the figure itself (e.g. when a black and white drawing of a horse is presented and the subject is asked questions such as: 'Is it an animal?', 'Is it dangerous?', 'Does it live at home?', etc.).

In its most severe form, the disturbance may become evident simply by observing a patient who, for example, uses some objects in an inappropriate manner or fails to recognize the object he is looking for. The patient described by Taylor & Warrington (1971) repeatedly complained about the lack of sugar in his tea despite the fact that the examiner continued to indicate the presence of a sugar bowl on the table in front of him. In this case, the patient was unable to use the sugar bowl because he could not recognize its functional properties.

The lesion responsible for associative agnosia is generally circumscribed to the occipito-temporal regions of the left hemisphere.

According to the model of Humphreys & Riddoch, associative agnosia consists of an inability to connect the output of a perceptive analysis made at the stage of object recognition with a more general underlying knowledge.

The existence of two storage areas (one for the structural knowledge of an object and the other for its semantic characteristics) has been confirmed by the study of patients with associative agnosia, some of whom had a preserved semantic and damaged presemantic store, and others vice versa. The former dissociation was demonstrated by Sartori & Job (Sartori & Job, 1988; Sartori *et al.*, 1992), who described a patient who could not do a test concerning the 'plausibility/reality' of a stimulus, or draw an object from memory, despite the fact that his functional and semantic knowledge was preserved. The patient gave correct answers to all of the questions concerning the environment in which certain animals live, the food they eat, and the fact that they were not wild animals, but could not give any kind of structural description, recognize them on the basis of a description provided by the examiner, or name them after their visual presentation.

The opposite disturbance (a preserved presemantic and a damaged semantic store) was found by Riddoch and Humphreys in patients who, although they managed to distinguish real from non-real objects, could not provide any reply to questions concerning their use, nor make any functional categorization when the stimuli were presented visually. The integrity of their knowledge of the perceptive structure allowed them to make correct judgements about the familiarity or otherwise of the stimuli, but not to recognize them. However, their semantic knowledge was preserved because they could reply correctly if they were given the name of the object verbally and asked to describe its use.

This particular disturbance has been called *semantic access agnosia* because, although semantic knowledge remains intact, it is not visually available.

One interesting aspect emerging from the study of Sartori & Job (1988) is the possibility that agnosic disturbances may be limited to only some semantic categories. The patients they described presented a deficit in the recognition of stimuli belonging to the category of foods and living things (animals, fruit and vegetables), but not in relation to non-living objects (clothes, furniture and means of transport). The opposite disturbance has also been observed (Warrington & McCarthy, 1987), although it is much rarer. The existence of a dual dissociation suggests that the information relating to the two semantic categories is processed in a different manner. Humphreys & Riddoch (1993) sustain that the greatest difficulties encountered by patients with associative agnosia for the categories of living things can be explained by the fact that their greater perceptive similarity requires a more profound analysis. However, although this interpretation is capable of explaining the behaviour of patients with a specific deficit in the structural knowledge of objects, in the case of those in which the disturbance affects the semantic store, it is necessary to hypothesize that the impairment lies exclusively at the level of semantic knowledge and is manifested regardless of whether the stimulus is presented visually or verbally (Silveri & Gainotti, 1988).

What has long been a matter of discussion in relation to associative agnosia is whether it is attributable to a deterioration in the traces deposited in the semantic store or the ability to gain access to the same. Shallice (1990) has proposed various criteria that can be used to make a differential diagnosis. Assuming an equal degree of disturbance, if the deficit is at the level of stimulus recognition, it should remain constant from test to test; if the problem is access, performances may vary from test to test. The hypothesis of access difficulties assumes that recognition should improve when the presentation is preceded by a 'primer' belonging to the same semantic category because, in this way, the category is pre-activated and this facilitates subsequent stimulus recognition. On the other hand, if the disturbance is due to a deterioration in the traces, recognition of an object should depend on its frequency of use. Prolonged stimulus presentation times favour performance in the case of an access disturbance, but have no effect if it is due to a deterioration in the traces.

Prosopagnosia

The term prosopagnosia, which was coined by Bodamer (Bodamer, 1947), refers to the inability to recognize the faces of known people, whose identification is preserved when it can be based on acoustic information (the voice) or non-physiognomic visual stimuli (the way of walking or dressing, or postural stance). In the milder forms, difficulties arise in relation to less well known people, particularly if they are encountered outside their usual context, or famous people even if patients sometimes retain a sense of familiarity. However, some very severe cases have also been reported: Hécaen & Angelergues (1962) described a patient who could not recognize his wife or even himself when he looked at the photograph taken on the day of his wedding. A prosopagnosic patient knows that a face is a face, and is generally able to state its sex and race, but he can no longer recognize it as 'that' face.

Two different explanations can be found in the literature. The first considers prosopagnosia to be a particular form of amnesia limited to the visual memory of perceptively similar stimuli (Damasio et al., 1982). According to this interpretation, which is mainly based on the cases reported by Damasio in which prosopagnosia was associated with other recognition difficulties, the disturbance reflects a general deficit in the ability to recognize an individual within a category (there is a description of a patient who simultaneously lost the ability to recognize human faces and different bird species).

The other interpretation is based on the dual dissociation between the ability to recognize faces and the ability to recognize the members of equally complex stimulus categories, and reflects a more modular conception of perceptive deficits. In this case, prosopagnosia is seen as a specific disturbance relating to the class 'faces'. Assal et al. (1984) described the case of a farmer who, although he had preserved the capacity to recognize familiar faces and those of famous people, he could no longer recognize his own cows. De Renzi (1986) reported the case of a patient with the opposite dissociation: a deficit in recognizing familiar faces in the absence of agnosia for other categories of stimuli.

In 1986, Bruce & Young developed a cognitive model to distinguish the various components underlying the complex ability to recognize faces. This model incorporates the majority of the data coming from neuropsychological research and studies of normal subjects concerning the

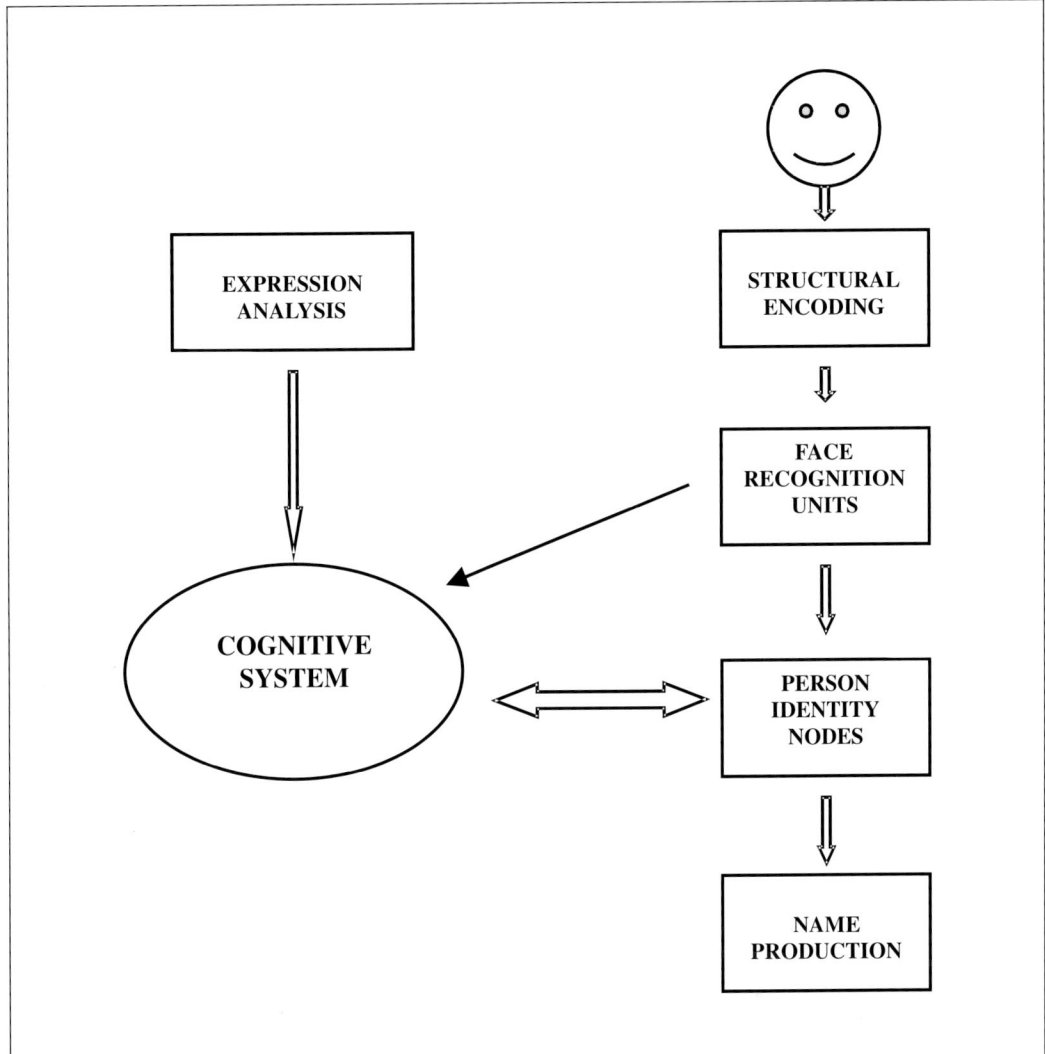

Fig. 1. Simplified version of the model of Bruce & Young (1986). Source: Denes & Pizzamiglio (1990).

processing of faces, and is capable of reconciling the two different positions mentioned above (Fig.1).

A first level of processing is *structural encoding*, which includes the representation of the face centred on the observer (who can therefore form different images depending on the viewing angle) and the more abstract, object-centred representation that summarizes the experiences we have had with it. A disturbance at this level will produce a deficit in the integration of the characteristics of a specific perceptive entity. Consequently, a patient will be unable to recognise faces seen from different angles or to decide whether two faces are the same or different.

At the next level, the abstract representation of the face is compared with the *face recognition unit*, a system that contains the perceptive structures of known faces. If there is concordance between the two types of information, a subject will be capable of recognizing a face as familiar, but can still not attribute it with a precise identity. A disturbance at this level means that a patient will be unable to distinguish known from unknown faces.

Real recognition takes place at the third level or personal identity node, which contains all of the semantic knowledge relating to the individual to whom the face belongs: his job, the circumstances in which we met him, his relationship with us, where he lives, and so on. Patients who have a disturbance at this level are incapable of providing information concerning the identity of a face and the semantic knowledge relating to it. De Haan et al. (1991) reported the case of a patient whose performances at structural encoding and the recognition of known faces were good, but who was totally incapable of providing any information relating to the faces recognized as being familiar.

The last level of analysis allows us to attribute a name to a previously recognized face. Selective disturbances at this level impede the recovery of the name belonging to a face that we recognize as known and about which we retain all of the related semantic information.

The hypothesis of a modular system underlying facial recognition makes it possible to suggest that some of the processes are the same as those allowing us to recognize objects, and that differentiation takes place at higher processing levels.

The results of neuropsychological research studies support the specificity of the class of faces in comparison with other forms of visual knowledge (Perret et al., 1987). It has been shown that the superior temporal sulcus of monkeys contains neurons that selectively discharge upon the presentation of faces: some cells are sensitive to certain parts of the face (eyes, mouth, hair), others to particular positions (full-face, profile, head down), and still others only respond to known faces (the face of the researcher, regardless of the position from which it is seen, its distance or its expression). These neurons may represent the anatomo-physiological substrate of the aroused face recognition units and support the thesis (Konorsky, 1967) that faces constitute a separate gnosic unit that may have developed during the course of evolution in order to encourage self-species recognition.

In man, the lesions responsible for prosopagnosia are circumscribed by the occipito-temporal border of the right hemisphere, although a clinically significant disturbance requires the involvement of both hemispheres.

Developmental agnosia

Very few studies refer to agnosic disturbances during the age of development, but it is not clear whether this is due to a tendency to neglect or misclassify this type of deficit, or the fact that it is really a rare condition. In 1968, Gordon reported the cases of two children affected by epileptic seizures who had difficulties in recognizing objects (Gordon, 1986). The first seems to be compatible with the description of simultanagnosia in adults: the child presented occipito-temporal EEG abnormalities and performed a recognition task adequately if the figures were presented individually, but not if more than one figure was presented at the same time. The other child presented bilateral occipital EEG abnormalities and had difficulty in recognizing large objects. However, neither of these cases seems to be a convincing example of object agnosia.

As far as face recognition is concerned, a large number of studies have described the development of this ability and the disturbances that may be encountered during the age of development.

Many of them have demonstrated that new-borns show a preference for faces over any other type of visual stimulus within the first few minutes of being born, which suggests that they already have some structural information available concerning facial characteristics. This information probably forms part of a primitive system related to the control of orientation (Johnson & Morton, 1991), which subsequently provides a stimulus for the development of the sophisticatedly complex adult mechanism described above. According to this interpretation (and in line with its cognitive viewpoint), cases of developmental prosopagnosia can be found whenever the development of face processing modules is impeded, a disturbance that may be associated with other deficits in visual analysis.

Another theory suggests that there is a region located around the upper temporal sulcus of the right hemisphere that is genetically programmed to process faces. Any damage or dysfunction in this area at birth or before could give rise to prosopagnosia in children (Campbell, 1992; De Haan & Campbell, 1991; McConachie, 1976; Temple, 1992). Recent neuroimaging studies (Mancini *et al.*, 1994) have shown that the presentation of faces (but not that of other visual stimuli) activates the temporal and infero-temporal cortex of 2-month-old new borns. Furthermore, face recognition seems to become a specialization of the right hemisphere as early as four months after birth.

The ability to recognize faces improves up to the age of ten years, and reaches the level of adult competence at about the age of 14 years. Despite the fact that there is no agreement among researchers concerning the progress of performance with age, it may be interesting to try to explain their main differences of opinion. Ellis & Flynn (1990) found that there is a significant difference between the performance of 7- and 10-year olds, and suggested that this is due to the greater amount of information that the older children can encode, as well as their better encoding strategies. This improvement may be due to the maturation or development of the aroused face recognition module, but it can also be interpreted as part of a more generalized perfecting of the executive memory processes that lead to an improvement in encoding strategies.

Two interesting cases of developmental prosopagnosia have been described (Campbell, 1992; De Haan & Campbell, 1991; McConachie, 1976; Temple, 1992), both of which can be interpreted using the model of Bruce & Young (1986) (Fig.1). The first concerns a 12-year-old girl (AB) whose neurological examination revealed nothing other than EEG abnormalities in the posterior part of the right hemisphere. The patient was first examined by McConachie in 1976, and subsequently evaluated as an adult by Campbell in 1992. AB has an average-superior intellectual level, shows no signs of any underlying deficit in perceptual functions, and is capable of distinguishing faces from non-faces; nevertheless, her ability to recognize known faces, analyse facial expressions and recognize objects is severely impaired. As far as the recognition of objects is concerned, her errors are based on their perceptive similarities and she has problems in identifying categorical examples that contain many perceptively similar stimuli. Furthermore, she has difficulties in recognizing objects seen from an unusual perspective. The interpretation of the authors suggests the existence of a disturbance at the level of structural encoding that has been present from birth and would explain the difficulties that the patient has in recognizing both faces and objects.

The second patient was described by Temple in 1992. Dr. S is a 60-year-old woman who says that she has always had difficulties in recognizing faces. The results of a neurological examination were negative, she has an above-average intellect, shows no signs of any underlying deficit in perceptive functions, and adequately performs tasks requiring object recognition or the structural encoding of faces (judgements concerning the age and sex of a face, and the recognition of an unknown face seen from different angles). Nevertheless, she is unable to distinguish famous from unknown faces, and has great difficulty in recovering semantic information relating to faces despite the fact that she can recover all of the information if she is told the name of the person concerned. The authors interpret these results by affirming that Dr. S may be an example of a person in whom the innate face processing module has been partially damaged. Her disturbance can be placed at a subsequent stage to that affecting AB: her structural encoding is intact and she is also capable of making an initial recording in face recognition units. Her problem is that she cannot preserve this information over time and/or use it to activate the nodes of personal identity.

Both of these cases involve a disturbance in face processing that is not related to any cerebral trauma, and so it is possible to define their deficit as congenital prosopagnosia. The differences between the two patients suggest that the various elements involved in face processing can be selectively damaged in congenital forms of the disturbance, as has already been demonstrated in the case of acquired forms.

References

Adler, A. (1950): Course and outcome of visual agnosia. *J. Nerv. Ment. Dis.* **111,** 41–51.

Assal, G., Faavre, C. & Anderes, J.P. (1984): Non reconnaissance d'animaux familiers chez un paysan. *Rev. Neurol.* **140,** 580–584.

Benton, A.L. & Hécaen, H. (1970): Stereoscopic vision in patients with unilateral cerebral disease. *Neurology* **20,** 1084–1088.

Bodamer, J. (1947): Die Prosopagnosie. *Archiv für Psychiatrie und Nervenkrankheiten* **179,** 6–53.

Bruce, V. & Young, A. (1986): Understanding face recognition. *Brit. J. Psychol.* **77,** 305–327.

Campbell, R. (1992): Face to face: interpreting a case of developmental prosopagnosia. In: *Mental lives: case studies in cognition*, ed. R. Campbell. Oxford: Basil Blackwell.

Campion, J. & Latto, R. (1985): Apperceptive agnosia due to carbon monoxide poisoning. An interpretation based on critical band masking from disseminated lesions. *Behav. Brain Res.* **15,** 227–240.

Damasio, A.R., Damasio, H., Van Hoesen, G.W. & Cornell, S. (1982). Prosopagnosia: anatomical basis and behavioural mechanisms. *Neurology* **32,** 331–341.

De Haan, E. & Campbell, R. (1991): A fifteen year follow-up of a case of developmental prosopagnosia. *Cortex* **27,** 489–509.

De Haan, E.H.F, Young, A.W. & Newcombe, F. (1991). A dissociation between the sense of familiarity and access to semantic information concerning familiar people. *Eur. J. Cognitive Psychol.* **3,** 51–57.

Denes, G. & Pizzamiglio, L. (1990): *Manuale di Neuropsicologia*. Bologna: Zanichelli.

De Renzi, E. (1986): Current issues on prosopagnosia. In: *Aspects of face processing*, eds. H.D. Ellis, M.A. Jeeves, F. Newcombe & A. Young, pp. 243–252. Dordrecht: Nijhoff.

De Renzi, E., & Spinnler, H. (1966): Facial recognition in brain damaged patients. *Neurology* **16,** 145–152.

De Renzi, E., Bonacini, M.G. & Faglioni, P. (1989): Right posterior brain damaged patients are poor at assessing the age of a face. *Neuropsychologia* **27,** 839–848.

Efron, R. (1968): What is perception? *Boston Studies in the Philosophy of Science* **4,** 137–173.

Ellis, H.D. & Flynn, R.H. (1990): Encoding and storage effects in 7-year-olds' and 10-year-olds' memory for faces. *Brit. J. Dev. Psychol.* **8,** 77–92.

Freud, S. (1891): *Zur Auffassung der Aphasien*. Vienna: Deuticke.

Gordon, N. (1968): Visual agnosia in childhood: VI. Preliminary communication. *Dev. Med. Child Neurol.* **10**, 377–379.

Hécaen, H. & Angelergues, R. (1962): Agnosia for faces (prosopagnosia). *Arch. Neurol.* **7**, 92–100.

Hécaen, H. & Angelergues, R. (1963): *La cécité psychique*. Paris: Masson.

Humphreys, G.W. & Riddoch, M.J. (1984): Routes to object constancy: implication from neurological impairments of object constancy. *Quart. J. Exp. Psychol.* **26A**, 385–415.

Humphreys, G.W. & Riddoch, M.J. (1987): The fractionation of visual agnosia. In: *Visual object processing: a cognitive approach*, eds. G.W. Humphreys & M.J. Riddoch. London: Erlbaum.

Humphreys, G.W. & Riddoch, M.J. (1993): Object agnosias. In: *Clinical neurology: international practice and research*, ed. C. Kennard. London: Baillière Tindall.

Johnson, M. & Morton, J. (1991): *Biology and cognitive development*. Oxford: Blackwell.

Konorsky, J. (1967): *Integrative activities of the brain: an interdisciplinary approach*. Chicago: University of Chicago Press.

Lissauer, H. (1890): Ein Fall von Seelenblindheit nebst einem Beitrag zur Theorie derselben. *Archiv Psychiatrie*, **21**, 222–270. Translated into English and reprinted In: *Lissauer on agnosia. Cognitive neuropsychology* (1988), vol. 5, ed. M. Jackson, pp. 155–192.

Mancini, J., de Schonen, S., Deruelle, C. & Massoulier, A. (1994): Face recognition in children with early right or left brain damage. *Develop. Med. Chld. Neurol.* **36**, 156–166.

Marr, D. (1980): Visual information processing: The structure and creation of visual representation. *Phil. Trans. Roy. Soc. (Lond.)*, **B290**, 199–218.

Marr, D. (1982): *Vision*. San Francisco: W.H. Freeman.

McConachie, H.R. (1976): Developmental prosopagnosia: a single case report. *Cortex* **12**, 76–82.

Perret, D.I., Mistlin, A.J. & Chitty, A.J., (1987): Visual neurons responsive to faces. *Trends Neurosci.* **10**, 358–364.

Sartori, G. & Job, R. (1988): The oyster with four legs: a neuropsychological study of the interaction of visual and semantic information. *Cognitive Neuropsychol.* **5**, 677–709.

Sartori, G., Job, R. & Coltheart, M. (1992): The neuropsychology of visual semantics. In: *Attention and performance*, vol. XIV, eds. D.E. Meyer & S. Kornblum. Hillsdale, NJ: Erlbaum.

Shallice, T. (1990): *From neuropsychology to mental structure*, Cambridge: Cambridge University Press, 1988. Italian edn. *Neuropsicologia e struttura della mente*. Bologna: Il Mulino.

Silveri, M.C. & Gainotti, G. (1988): Interaction between vision and language in category specific impairment. *Cognitive Neuropsychol.* **5**, 677–709.

Taylor, A. & Warrington, E.K. (1971): Visual agnosia: a single case report. *Cortex* **7**, 152–161.

Temple, C.M. (1992): Developmental memory impairment: faces and patterns. In: *Mental lives: case studies in cognition*, ed. R. Campbell, pp. 199–215. Oxford: Basil Blackwell.

Warrington, E.K. (1985): Agnosia: the impairment of object recognition. In: *Handbook of clinical neurology, clinical neuropsychology*, vol. 1 (45), ed. J.A.M. Frederiks. Amsterdam: Elsevier Science Publishers.

Warrington, E.K. & James, M. (1988): Visual apperceptive agnosia: a clinico-anatomical study. *Cortex* **24**, 13–32.

Warrington, E.K. & McCarthy, R.A. (1987): Categories of knowledge: further fractionation and an attempted integration. *Brain* **110**, 1273–1296.

Warrington, E.K. & Taylor, A.M. (1973): The contribution of the right parietal lobe to object recognition. *Cortex* **9**, 152–164.

Chapter 11

Language in children with early brain damage: the development of brain-behaviour relations

Judy Snitzer Reilly

Laboratory for Infant and Child Studies, San Diego State University, 6363 Alvarado Ct #221, San Diego, CA 92120, USA

In the last twenty years or so, new technologies have permitted us to 'look' inside the human brain to better understand its functioning. However, brain-behaviour relationships have long been of interest to the scientific community. In the domain of language, Paul Broca's discovery in the 1860s that the left frontal cortex was implicated in productive language and Carl Wernicke's subsequent studies revealing the left temporal lobe to be critical for language comprehension were landmark events. Moreover, their findings have been confirmed by numerous studies for a wide range of languages (for a review, see Goodglass, 1993) including American Sign Language (Poizner et al., 1987). Interestingly, in the last 25 years or so, the right hemisphere has also been implicated in aspects of linguistic processing, especially in discourse and non-literal uses of language (e.g. Brownell et al., 1990, VanLancker & Kempler, 1986, Gardner et al., 1983; Hough, 1990; Joanette et al., 1990; Kaplan et al., 1990). At present we have an extensive body of research on those structures mediating adult language functions, but we are only beginning to understand how these relationships develop in children.

In the 1930s Margaret Kennard conducted studies of young and infant monkeys and found recovery of motor function after early lesions (Kennard, 1936). In the realm of language, Lenneberg (1967) found that children with early onset strokes do not suffer the same irreversible damage as adults with homologous lesions. Together these findings raised the possibility that children's brains, unlike those of adults, are flexible and reflect a wider potential for assuming diverse behavioural functions. According to the strongest view of this hypothesis of equipotentiality, any area of the brain could assume responsibility for any behavioural function. Lenneberg also suggested that the plasticity, or flexibility, responsible for this broad potential decreased substantially by adolescence when the brain had lateralized, and different cortical areas had assumed responsibility for specific behavioural functions. In the ensuing years, additional studies in children with brain damage have noted subtle yet persistent language deficits in children with early brain damage. Reviews have been written by a number of researchers, including Hécaen, 1976; Riva & Cazzaniga, 1986; Vargha-Khadem et al., 1992; Aram, 1988, 1991, and most recently, Eisele & Aram, 1994, 1995. Studies of children with hemispherectomies (e.g. Dennis & Whitaker, 1976; Dennis & Kohn, 1975; Vargha-Khadem et al., 1991) have also been instructive in this discovery process. While all of these studies have contributed to our understanding of language functions in children with neurological dysfunction, many have included children who incurred damage at different ages, and these studies have come to differing conclusions regarding the nature and role of the left hemisphere in language development. Our goal over the last ten years has been to understand the development of brain-language relations from the beginning of life by following the course of language development in children with early unilateral focal brain damage. All of the children in this group suffered their cerebral insult before six months of age, that is, pre-linguistically. By prospectively chronicling their language development from infancy to adolescence, we can begin to address the following basic questions:

(1) Localization of function

- To what degree is language specified early on? Do behavioural patterns correlate with site of brain damage? Are they comparable to those of adults with homologous injuries?

(2) Neuroplasticity

- Do behavioural deficits persist or is there recovery of function over time?
- Does the deficit express itself differentially over time?

(3) The nature of the language acquisition process

- How flexible is the language acquisition process itself? Is the process fairly rigid or are there many ways to approach learning a language?

In the remainder of the chapter, I will first present an overview of the developmental milestones for language development in typically developing children, as background. Then, as a prelude to a discussion of our studies on narrative, I will summarize the studies on early language development in this special population. The chapter will then centre on later language development in these children with early focal brain damage in the context of narrative discourse as narratives will permit us to examine those aspects of language mediated by both the left and right hemispheres in adults.

Language development in typically developing children

For the past thirty years, a broad base of studies has examined early language development in children from a variety of languages and across a wide array of language families. The findings are consistent: children acquire languages in principled ways (e.g. Slobin, 1985). Although specific features characterize the acquisition of particular languages, researchers have identified a set of milestones that children pass through as they grapple with learning their native tongue. The following table presents a sketch of these developmental milestones with examples in both English and Italian. It is important to note that the ages of acquisition for particular structures are provided only as a guide, since researchers have found extensive variability in the timing of normal language development (Fenson et al., 1993).

With this general picture of the sequence of language development in typically developing children as a backdrop, we are ready to review the studies of the first stages of language acquisition in children with early unilateral brain damage.

Table 1. Language milestones

Milestone	Age of onset	Examples
Word comprehension	8–10 months	
Single word production (often accompanied by gestures)	11–13 months	Luce. Guarda. Allgone. Doggie.
Word combinations	20–24 months	Mamma latte. Want cookie.
Morphology	24–28+ months	Bimbi giocano. Two socks.
Complex sentences	36+ months	Nonna piange 'che il bimbo va via. Chrissy's crying cuz h'es sad.
Connected discourse	42+ months	–

Early language development in children with focal brain injury

The group of children that have participated in the following studies all suffered a unilateral focal cerebral insult either pre- or perinatally; the lesions have all been confirmed by CT scan or MRI before the child reached six months of age, that is, before they have acquired any language. Additionally, these children were free from other birth complications that might suggest more diffuse brain damage.

With respect to their early language development, as a group, these children are delayed in both comprehension and production of first words (Bates *et al.*, 1997). That is, regardless of side of lesion, the children with focal brain damage are delayed when compared to their age and gender matched controls. There is sufficient variability in the group that some children are within the normal range of performance. Nonetheless, as a whole, children with either right hemisphere damage (RHD) or left hemisphere damage (LHD) are delayed in the onset of language. Within this overall delay, there are interesting and unexpected site-specific behaviour patterns. In studies using parental report as a means to assess early comprehension and production skills, Bates and her colleagues presented cross-sectional data from over 50 toddlers with unilateral brain damage (Bates *et al.*, 1997) which confirmed the earlier findings of Thal *et al.*, (1991) which included a smaller cohort. Both studies showed that in children from 10–17 months, infants with right posterior damage were more delayed in comprehension than the rest of the focal lesion (FL) children. Bates also found that toddlers (from 19–31 months) with either left or right frontal damage were more delayed in production than would be expected, but this was a transient effect. Finally, looking at both parental report and spontaneous speech data in children from 20 to 44 months, children with left temporal damage evidenced more delays in productive vocabularies and had shorter utterances than the rest of the FL group, and the group as a whole continued to perform significantly below controls.

In summary, from these studies of early language development in this population, we have seen that the children with early brain damage lagged behind their controls on measures of comprehension, production, and mean length of utterance. In addition to the overall delay for the group as a whole, an additional and unpredicted lag was found in the younger children with right posterior damage for comprehension and a persistent delay in vocabulary and then in morphology, as measured by mean length of utterance (MLU) was found in children with left temporal damage. Neither of these patterns maps onto the adult profile for brain organization of language which would have predicted that children with right hemisphere damage would have shown normal language development; those with left frontal damage would have evidenced production delays; and those with posterior left damage would have demonstrated impaired comprehension. Overall, the findings suggest that initially, at least, both hemispheres are implicated in *initiating* the language acquisition process, and that rather than being localized to the left hemisphere, as is true for the vast majority of adults, language as it is being acquired is a rather broadly distributed function.

Narratives

Once children are producing sentences and are well along in mastering the basic morphological structures of their language, linguistic development involves developing more sophisticated discourse skills and using particular syntactic structures with increasing frequency and effectiveness. Beginning at about age three and a half to four years, we see an increasing ability to recruit particular linguistic structures for specific discourse purposes, e.g. to provide clearer directions, relate more coherent stories, to tell better jokes. In light of this developmental transition, researchers have used narratives to investigate multiple aspects of language and discourse in preschool and school age children who are typically developing (Petersen & McCabe, 1983; Bamberg, 1987; Stein & Glenn, 1982; Berman & Slobin, 1994; Bamberg and Marchman, 1990) as well as atypical populations (e.g. Reilly *et al.*, 1990; Dennis & Lovett, 1990; Tager-Flusberg, 1994, 1995). The goal of the narrative studies to be presented below is twofold: first, to follow the progress of language development in the children with focal brain damage through school age, and secondly to use narratives as a context to evaluate both the core structural aspects of language mediated by the left hemisphere in adults as well as those in which the right hemisphere in adults is also implicated, e.g. emotion words and story coherence. We will focus on the development of narratives in children from 4–11 years old and include 30 children with FL (18 with LHD and 13 with RHD) and their age and gender matched controls (Reilly *et al.*, 1998).

In our narrative task, the child looked through wordless picture book, *Frog, where are you?* (Mayer, 1979) and then with the book available, told the story to the experimenter. The story is about a boy and his dog who had found a frog and put him in a jar. During the night, when the boy had fallen asleep, the frog escaped. The subsequent episodes include the boy's search for the frog and his adventures during the quest. The search concludes with the discovery of a frog, his mate and a clutch of babies. In the end, the boy takes one of the baby frogs and returns home with his dog.

As noted earlier, the pre- and perinatal strokes are structurally similar to those suffered by adults later in life. According to the adult model, we would expect a child with LHD to have problems with morphology and syntax whereas those aspects of language would be spared in children with RHD. In contrast, those with RHD would be expected to make fewer inferences, and show problems with discourse coherence. After the stories were transcribed, we looked at those aspects of the narratives which were predicted to differentially affect the groups according to the adult model. Table 2 below presents those aspects of language and narratives in which one might expect deficits according to the adult model.

Table 2. Predictions from the adult model

Narrative coding for presumed left hemisphere functions

Propositions: Length of the story as assessed by number of story related propostions

Morphological errors: Include both errors of omission and commission, e.g. determiners, auxiliaries
– An' the dog -O- being chased from a bees.
(TARGET: And the dog is being chased by the bees.)

Complex sentences: Coordinate and Subordinate clauses; Verb complements, within a sentence boundary
– The boy was lookin' in the hole and the dog was barking at the bees.
– When he woke up, the boy was gone.
– He climbed up the tree to see if the frog was inside.

Narrative coding for presumed right hemisphere functions

Story components: The story includes eight episodes including:
– Setting
– Initiating event
– Five search episodes
– Resolution

Narrative theme:

     Explicit mention (looking for or calling the lost frog)
– They're being quiet to see if the frog's in there.
– He's looking for his frog.
     Reiteration of theme:
– He looked in the tree, but the frog wasn't there.

Lexical evaluation: Include evaluative words, e.g. emotional labels, intensifiers; causal words and mental verbs.
– An' the dog's <u>scaring</u> the bees.
– An' he was <u>tryin'</u> to find the frog.
– An' the boy was <u>callin' for</u> his frog.

The children's stories

Our first finding was that the children with FL tell shorter stories than the control children; overall, they talk less than their typically developing peers, however, there was no difference according to side of lesion. In addition to shorter stories, that is, fewer overall propositions or clauses, as a group, the younger FL children include fewer story episodes than their controls. Again, this was true for both RHD and LHD groups; there was no effect for lesion site. However, in the older group (ages 7–10 years) there were no differences between the clinical and neurologically intact group with respect to the completeness of their narratives, suggesting that, although shorter, the stories of the children with brain damage (either RHD or LHD) still include the relevant narrative components.

LOCALIZATION OF BRAIN LESIONS AND DEVELOPMENTAL FUNCTIONS

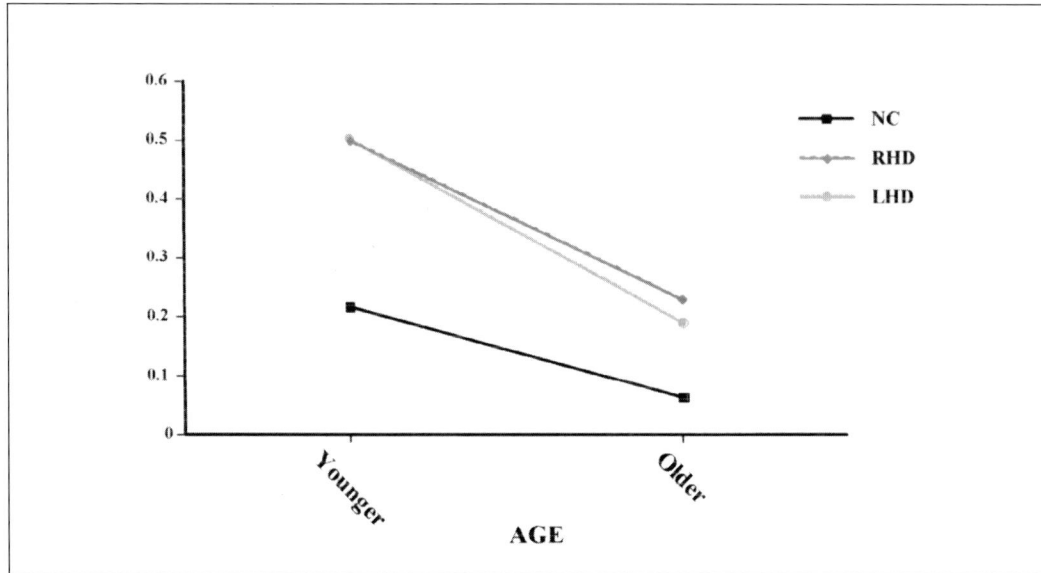

Fig. 1. Proportion of morphological errors.

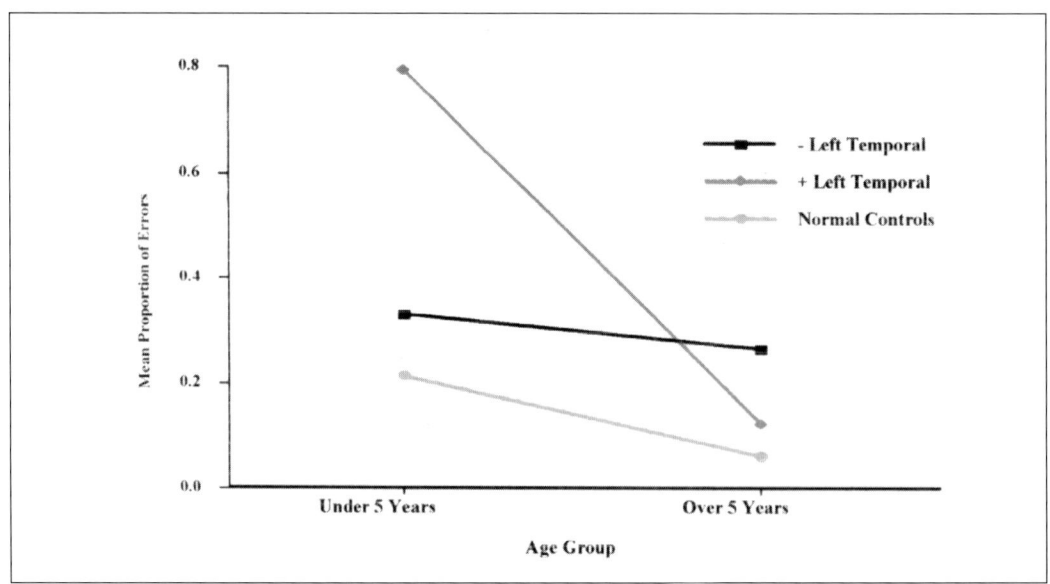

Fig. 2. Proportion of morphological errors and presence/absence of left temporal damage.

Putative left hemisphere functions

Grammatical morphology

Although English is not a language rich in grammatical morphology, it nonetheless poses a challenge for children acquiring English, and it is not until age five that typically developing children have substantially mastered English grammatical morphology. Errors in this domain are both of commission and omission. Both determiners and the copula are candidates for omission (e.g. '*0* boy and *0* dog *0* walking home' rather than the target 'The boy and the dog were walking home'). Commission errors tend to be in tense marking ('he *singed*' rather than 'he sang') and agreement on verbs ('she *were* running' rather than 'she was running') and pronominal agreement ('*him* likes ice cream' rather than 'he likes ice cream'). Our findings in this area were consonant with the previous studies in the children with early brain insults. Overall, as a group, the younger FL children (ages 4–6) made many more errors than controls; however, by age seven or so, they were performing in the normal range. Interestingly, when we compared the frequency of morphological errors of those children with LHD against those with RHD, there was no difference. In fact their profiles were identical (see Fig. 1).

However, as in the Bates *et al.* (1997) study, if we compared those with left temporal damage with all the other children in the FL group without left temporal damage, i.e. children with RHD or left posterior damage, the four younger children who constitute the left temporal group are significantly more delayed in morphology than the rest of the FL group. Note also that this difference is resolved in the older group (Fig. 2). Because the younger group with left temporal damage included only four children, this result must be viewed with caution, but the findings are consonant with the earlier studies and do not map onto our adult generated predictions.

An interesting point to note here is that for the children with focal brain damage, the quality of the errors is similar to those of normal children as in the following examples:

Table 3. Examples of morphological errors

(NC 4;1):	He's waiting by *hisselfl*
(NC 3;6):	He *0* mad *of* the dog/
(NC 4;0):	The dog jumped out here and *finded* the rock/
(RHD 4;6):	The dog *0* licking *0* in the face/
(LHD 5;0):	Then they *seed* the two frogs again.
(LHD 6;1):	*Him* went and *him* ran/
(RHD 7;1):	Ouch he said to the boy to *hisselfl*

Moreover, if we look at the frequency of errors in typically developing three and four year olds, they are similar in number to those of the brain damaged children at five and six. In sum, it appears that regardless of lesion site, the children with brain damage are delayed in the acquisition of grammatical morphology, and that the process of acquisition, as judged by the type of grammatical errors, is similar to typically developing children. These qualitative similarities suggest that both the typically developing children and those with early cerebral insults are approaching the language learning task in a similar fashion. The atypical finding appears to be in timing, rather than in quality. However, we must also keep in mind that English is not rich morphologically and therefore the kinds of errors one might make are rather limited. Because Italian is a language very rich in grammatical morphology, in our future work with our Italian colleagues we will be in a position to address this issue by investigating the language acquisition in Italian children with early strokes.

Complex syntax

Anyone can tell a story using only simple sentences, and their story would be grammatically correct. In this case, however, it becomes the responsibility of the addressee to make inferences about the relationships of events encoded in these individual clauses. In contrast, if the narrator

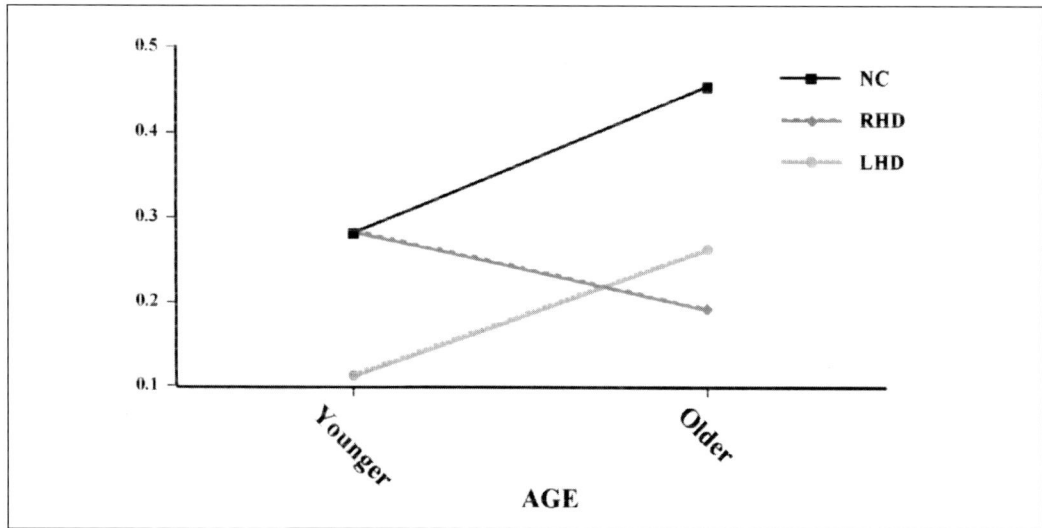

Fig. 3. Frequency of complex syntax. Proportion of morphological errors.

uses complex sentences, especially those with subordinate clauses, the storyteller makes the relationship between clauses explicit. For example, one might say, 'The boy went to sleep. The frog escaped.' Or, if one wanted to clarify the temporal relationship between these events, one could say, 'While the boy was sleeping, the frog escaped'. These subordinate clause conjunctions, in addition to the aspect marker on the verb (perfect or progressive), are the linguistic mechanisms which integrate the events of the story.

When we looked at the use of complex sentences in the narratives (as seen in Fig. 3) we found that for the control children, as they develop through the school age period, they use increasingly complex sentences in their stories and they also use more types of sentences as they get older. In fact, whereas the younger children favour the semantically broad '*and*' as a connective, the older children are using many more semantically specific subordinators, e.g. '*because*', '*since*', '*when*'. Recall that we hypothesized that the children with LHD would be particularly affected in this domain. In contrast to our original expectations, we found that they follow the normal trajectory but at a slower rate, and at the oldest data point, their performance is within the normal range. Surprisingly, it is the children with RHD who show an unexpected profile: from the first to the second data point, their profile is relatively flat. We have recently looked at longitudinal data from eight of the children with LHD and eight more with RHD. Initially, those with RHD also show this flat profile and only in the later school years do they demonstrate a significant increase in the use of complex sentences. Because complex sentences are the mechanism to link episodes of the story together, we have speculated that this plateau on the part of the children with RHD may reflect a broader integrative deficit, similar to that identified by Stiles in her studies of spatial analysis in this same group of children (Stiles & Nass, 1991; Stiles *et al.*, 1998).

Putative right hemisphere functions

Recall that whereas our hypotheses for the children with LHD concerned core language structures, for those with RHD, the adult model would predict that they would have more problems with lexical evaluation and extracting the theme of the story.

Evaluative devices

Evaluation is that aspect of a story that incorporates the narrator's perspective on the events that constitute the plot. Labov & Waletzsky (1967) introduced the notion of evaluation to characterize the clauses in the narrative that commented on and stopped the temporal flow of the referential clauses that are the plot of the story. We have extended their idea to include both linguistic and paralinguistic devices that reflect the narrator's point of view (Reilly *et al.,* 1990; Bamberg & Damrad-Frye, 1991; Losh *et al.,* 1999). Evaluation brings life and interest to a story; for example, evaluative devices include the lexically encoded inferences regarding emotions and cognitions of characters, direct quotes from the characters, intensifiers (e.g. *really, very*), as well as expressions that convey degrees of certainty (e.g. *probably, might*). Preschoolers often use prosody to fulfill this function, and these devices are used infrequently in kindergartners. However, their use increases during school age, and adults can use them quite skillfully (Reilly, 1992; Bamberg & Reilly, 1996). In this sense, lexically encoded evaluation might be considered a later development, or an optional component, like icing on a cake. In our typically developing group, we see children using increasing numbers of evaluative devices as they get older. The children with FL are significantly below normal, although children in the FL group recruit them more frequently with age.

In addition to the linguistic structures that children use, we were also interested in how they constructed their stories. We envisage a story as a temporally organized sequence of events with an overarching theme (in this case, the search) which binds the events together, and in this case, motivates the boy's behaviour in the individual episodes. To capture these narrative dimensions, we analysed this domain by ascertaining the completeness of their stories by coding the events they included and examining the degree to which they made explicit the theme of the story: 'The boy is searching for the frog.' Again, we hypothesized that RHD children would have more difficulty with these aspects of the narrative than those with LHD or normals. Contrary to our expectations, there were no significant differences and all groups improved with age. That is, all the children mentioned more and more episodes with age. Moreover, they also mentioned that the boy was looking for the frog, and as they got older, they began to integrate the individual episodes with the overarching search theme, as in, 'He looked into the hole in the tree to see if the frog was there'. However, the lesion group did so significantly less frequently than controls. Given these findings overall, it appears that the children with RHD do not have significant problems with forming these types of inferences. The protracted delay in their use of complex syntax, noted earlier, suggests that the problem may reside in recruiting the appropriate syntactic form to convey and explicitly link those relationships, rather than in inferring the relationships themselves.

So to summarize our findings:

(1) All groups improve over time (children with brain damage display a similar profile to younger controls)

(2) RHD and LHD generally pattern together and perform similarly to normals by middle childhood.

(3) Errors committed by the clinical group are similar to those committed by normally developing children.

With these data in mind, we can return to address our original questions:

Our first question concerned the degree to which language is localized from an early point in development. We found that the language profiles of the children with focal brain damage do not map onto those of adults with comparable damage. In fact, irrespective of damage site, the children show initial delay, and subsequent development. Hence, although perhaps not optimally suited for language, our data suggest that multiple areas of the brain can subserve language functions. Additionally the data suggest that the brain areas suited to acquire language may be more broadly distributed than those necessary to maintain language functioning once it has been acquired.

Regarding the issue of neuroplasticity, the fairly rapid acquisition of the morphosyntax of English in the children with early brain damage *regardless of lesion site* is strong evidence of the flexibility of the developing brain. In those morphosyntactic structures that we examined, we found that for the mandatory grammatical functions, the children in the FL group were initially delayed, but eventually performing within the normal range. However, we do not know the extent of this plasticity, that is, we do not know whether they will continue to expand their syntactic repertoire to acquire some of the optional, but more adult-like morphological and syntactic forms.

Finally, with respect to the nature of the language acquisition process itself, the finding that the morphological errors of all the groups of children are of the same types, that is, that the differences are in quantity rather than in quality, suggests that the language acquisition process itself is fairly rigid in nature. Additionally, the slope of the trajectory for the FL children for morphology is similar to younger developing preschoolers. It appears that once children begin to acquire grammatical morphemes, the rate and nature of the acquisition processes are similar; what differs is when you begin. In sum, developmental differences appear to be in timing rather than in kind.

In this chapter we have presented an overview of language development in children with early focal brain damage as a means to understand the development of the brain-bases for language and the flexibility of the developing brain. Together our findings have shown that, overall, children with brain damage are delayed in the acquisition of language, regardless of side of lesion, but eventually do go on to acquire the lexicon and grammar and be competent speakers of English. As we look over the children's stories, it is clear that just as different aspects of language develop at different points in time so, too, do the deficits change over time. In sum, language development continues in the face of early unilateral brain damage, and although recruiting alternative neural means, the children with early focal brain damage follow a similar, but delayed, behavioural path to their typically developing counterparts.

Acknowledgement: This resaerch was supported by NINDS-NIH Grant P50–NS–22343 and NIDCD P01 DC 01289–029.

References

Aram, D. (1988): Language sequelae of unilateral brain lesions in children. In: *Language, communication and the brain*, ed. F. Plum, pp. 171–197. New York: Raven Press.

Aram, D. (1991): Review of language development in children with focal brain injury. Paper presented to the Venice Conference on Developmental Neuropsychology, Venice (San Servolo). (Published in Italian in: *Neuropsicologia in età evolutiva*, eds. D. Riva, A. Benton & H. Levin. Milan: Franco Angeli.

Bamberg, M. (1987): *The acquisition of narratives*. Berlin: Mouton de Gruyter.

Bamberg, M. & Damrad-Frye, R. (1991): On the ability to provide evaluative comments: further explorations of children's narrative competencies. *J. Child Lang.* **18,** 689–710.

Bamberg, M. & Marchman, V. (1990): What holds a narrative together? The linguistic encoding of episode boundaries. *Papers in Pragmatics* **4,** 58–121.

Bamberg, M. & Reilly, J.S. (1996): Emotion, narrative and affect. In: *Social interaction, social context and language,* eds. D.I. Slobin, J. Gerhardt, A. Kyratzis & J. Guo. Essays in Honor of Susan Ervin-Tripp. Norwood, NJ: Lawrence Erlbaum Associates.

Bates, E.A.,Thal, D., Trauner, D., Fenson, J., Aram, D., Eisele, J. & Nass, R. (1997): From first words to grammar in children with focal brain injury. *Dev. Neuropsychol.* **13,** 275–343.

Berman, R. & Slobin, D.I. (1994): *Relating events in narrative.* Hillsdale, NJ: Lawrence Erlbaum Associates.

Brownell, H., Simpson, T., Bihrle, A., Potter, H. & Gardner, H. (1990): Appreciation of metaphoric alternative word meanings by left and right brain-damaged patients. *Neuropsychologia* **28,** 375–384.

Dennis, M. & Kohn, B. (1975): Comprehension of syntax in infantile hemiplegics after cerebral hemidecortication. *Brain Lang.* **2,** 472–482.

Dennis, M. & Whitaker, H.A. (1976): Language acquisition following hemidecortication: linguistic superiority of the left over the right hemisphere. *Brain Lang.* **3,** 404–433.

Eisele, J. & Aram, D. (1994): Comprehension and imitation of syntax following early hemisphere damage. *Brain Lang.* **46,** 212–231.

Eisele, J. & Aram, D. (1995): Lexical and grammatical development in children with early hemisphere damage: a cross-sectional view from birth to adolescence. In: *Handbook of child language,* eds. P. Fletcher & B. MacWhinney. Oxford: Basil Blackwell.

Fenson, L., Dale, P., Reznick, J.S., Thal, D., Bates, E., Hartung, J., Peyhick, S. & Reilly, J. (1993): *MacArthur communicative inventories: user's guide and manual.* San Diego, CA: Singular Publishing Group.

Gardner, H., Brownell, H., Wapner, W. & Michelow, D. (1983): Missing the point: the role of the right hemisphere in the processing of complex linguistic materials. In: *Cognitive processing in the right hemisphere,* ed. E. Perceman. New York: Academic Press.

Goodglass, H. (1993): *Understanding aphasia.* San Diego, CA: Academic Press.

Hécaen, H. (1976): Acquired aphasia in children and the ontogenesis of hemispheric functional specialization. *Brain Lang.* **3,** 114–134.

Hough, M. (1990): Narrative comprehension in adults with right and left hemisphere brain damage: theme organization. *Brain Lang.* **38,** 253–277.

Joanette, Y., Goulet, P. & Hannequin, D. (1990): *Right hemisphere and verbal communication.* New York: Springer-Verlag.

Kaplan, J., Brownell, H., Jacobs, J. & Gardner, H. (1990): The effects of right hemisphere damage on the pragmatic interpretation of conversational remarks. *Brain Lang.* **38,** 315–333.

Labov, W. & Waletzky, J. (1967): Narrative analysis: oral versions of personal experience. In: *Essays on the verbal and visual arts,* ed. J. Helm. Seattle: University of Washington Press.

Kennard, M. (1936): Age and other factors in motor recovery from precentral lesions in monkeys. *Am. J. Physiol.* **115,** 138–146.

Lenneberg, E.H. (1967): *Biological foundations of language.* New York: Wiley.

Losh, M., Bellugi, U., Reilly, J. & Anderson, D. (1999). The integrity and independence of evaluation in narrative: evidence from children with Williams Syndrome.

Mayer, M. (1979): *Frog, where are you?* New York: Dial Press.

Peterson, C. & McCabe, E. (1983): *Developmental psycholinguistics: three ways of looking at a child's narrative.* New York: Plenum Press.

Poizner, H., Klima, E. & Bellugi, U. (1987): *What the hands reveal about the brain.* Cambridge, MA.: MIT/Bradford Books.

Reilly, J.S. (1992): How to tell a good story: the intersection of language and affect in children's narrative. *J. Narrative Life Hist.* **2,** 355–377.

Reilly, J. Bates, E. & Marchman, V. (1998): Narrative discourse in children with early focal brain damage. *Brain Lang.* **61,** 335–375.

Reilly, J., Klima, E. & Bellugi, U. (1990): Once more with feeling: affect and language in atypical populations. *Dev. Psychopathol.* **2 (4),** 367–391.

Riva, D. & Cazzaniga, L. (1986): Late effects of unilateral brain lesions sustained before and after age one. *Neuropsychologia* **24,** 423–428.

Slobin, D.I. (1985): *The crosslinguistic study of language acquisition.* Hillsdale, NJ: Lawrence Erlbaum Associates.

Stein, N.L. & Glenn, C. (1982): Children's concept of time: the development of a story schema. In: *The developmental psychology of time*, ed. W.J. Friedman. New York: Academic Press.

Stiles, J. & Nass, R. (1991): Spatial grouping activity in young children with congenital right or left hemisphere brain injury. *Brain Cognition* **15,** 201–222.

Stiles, J., Bates, E.A., Thal, D., Trauner, D. & Reilly, J.S. (1998): Linguistic, cognitive and affective development in children with pre- and peri-natal focal brain injury: a ten year overview from the San Diego longitudinal project. In: *Advances in infancy research*, vol. 12, eds. C. Rovee-Collier, L. Lipsitt & H. Hayne.

Tager-Flusberg, H. (1994): Dissociations in form and function in the acquisition of language by autistic children. In: *Constraints on language acquisition: studies of atypical children,* ed. H. Tager-Flusberg, pp. 175–194. Hillsdale, NJ: Lawrence Erlbaum.

Tager-Flusberg, H. (1995): 'Once upon a ribbit': stories narrated by autistic children. *Br. J. Dev. Psychol.* **13,** 45–59.

Thal, D.J., Marchman, V.A., Stiles, J., Aram, D., Trauner, D., Nass, R. & Bates, E. (1991): Early lexical development in children with focal brain injury. *Brain Lang.* **40,** 491–527.

VanLancker, D. & Kempler, D. (1986): Comprehension of familiar phrases by left- but not by right-hemisphere-damaged patients. *Brain Lang.* **32,** 265–277.

Vargha-Khadem, F., Isaacs, E., Papleoudi, H., Polkey, C. & Wilson, J. (1991): Development of language in six hemispherectomized patients. *Brain* **114,** 473–495.

Vargha-Khadem, F. & Polkey, C.E. (1992): A review of cognitive outcome after hemidecortication in humans. In: *Recovery from brain damage: Advances in experimental medicine and biology*, eds. F.D. Rosen & D.A. Johnson, **325,** pp. 137–171. New York: Plenum Press.

Chapter 12

Non-verbal learning disabilities: development of the syndrome and the model

Byron P. Rourke

Department of Psychology, University of Windsor, Windsor, Ontario Canada N9B 3P4
Child Study Center, Yale University, New Haven, CT, USA

Summary

In this chapter, the background of the investigative effort that has been expended in our laboratory is presented. Then, the fruits of this endeavour are examined within the context of the models that we have constructed to explain these data. In all of this, the principal point to bear in mind (given the 'right hemisphere' focus of this section) is the following: we view the significant disruption of right hemispheral systems in children (and, in some cases, adults) to be a *sufficient* condition for the appearance of the syndrome of non-verbal learning disabilities (NLD). At the same time, it is clear that aetiologies that involve *direct* disruption of right hemispheral systems are not *necessary* for the exhibition of the syndrome. This distinction should become clear as we proceed.

Historical overview

Since 1971, we have engaged in the intensive investigation of two subtypes of children with learning disabilities (LD). As a result of our clinical observations and empirical investigations, we are able to state with considerable confidence the characteristics (content validity) of the two subtypes, as follows.

Basic phonological processing disorder (BPPD)

Children of this subtype exhibit many relatively poor psycholinguistic skills in conjunction with well-developed assets in visual–spatial–organizational, tactile–perceptual, psychomotor, and non-verbal problem-solving skills. They perform very poorly in single-word reading and spelling and significantly better, though still impaired, in mechanical arithmetic. Their outstanding problem is in the area of phonological awareness and processing. The model (content and developmental dynamics) that we have developed to encompass these observations and research findings is outlined in Fig. 1.

It should be emphasized that the patterns of academic deficits experienced by individuals who

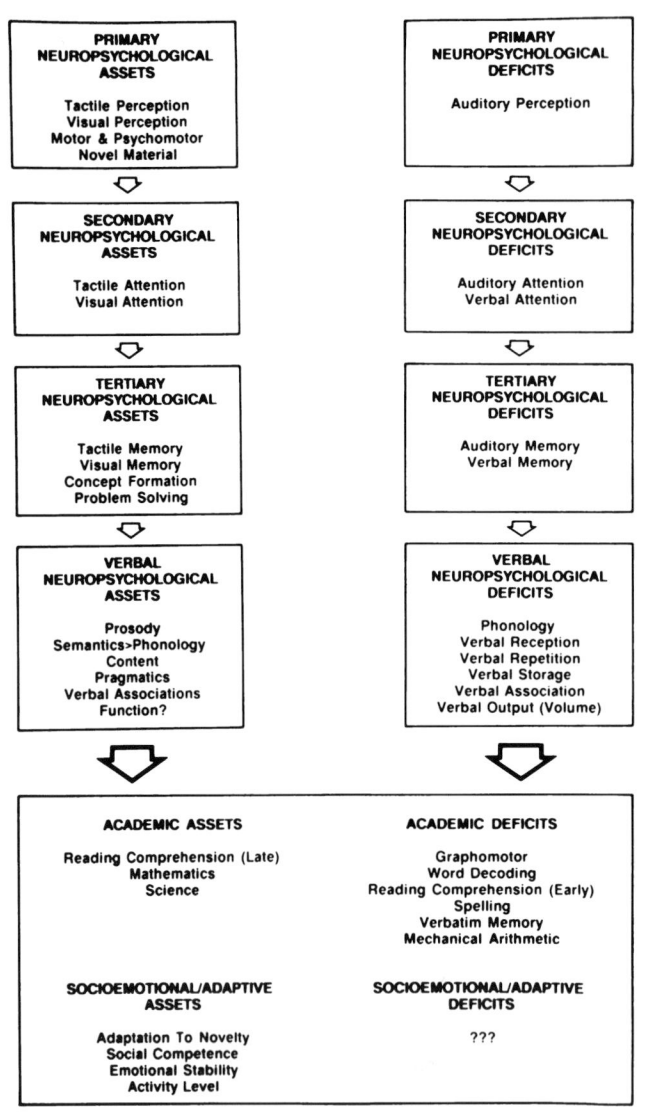

Fig. 1. Content and dynamics of basic phonological processing disorder.

exhibit this subtype of LD are viewed as the *direct* result of the interaction of the primary, secondary, tertiary, and linguistic neuropsychological assets and deficits that are outlined in Fig. 1. For example, considering the hypothesized 'deficit' stream, the primary neuropsychological deficits experienced by the child with BPPD are seen as having to do with aspects of auditory perception. These deficits relate especially to phonemic awareness and processing (discrimination, segmentation and blending). Such deficits would be expected to eventuate in disordered attention to auditory–verbal input; in turn, problems in memory for verbal material delivered through the auditory modality would be expected to ensue. This set of deficits would be expected to eventuate in the particular set of linguistic deficiencies outlined in Fig. 1. It is clear that the pattern of neuropsychological assets and deficits exhibited by persons with BPPD would be most consistent with dysfunction of some systems within the left cerebral hemisphere.

The academic and psychosocial/adaptive deficiencies listed are the expected sequelae of these neuropsychological deficits. It is especially important to note that this set of neuropsychological deficits is not expected to lead, in a necessary way, to an increased frequency, or any particular configuration, of problems in psychosocial/adaptive behaviour either within or without the academic situation (Rourke, 1988a, 1989; Rourke & Fuerst, 1992). For a fuller description of BPPD, the interested reader is referred to Rourke (1989).

Non-verbal learning disabilities (NLD)

Persons with the other subtype – which we refer to as the NLD syndrome – exhibit outstanding neuropsychological deficits in visual–spatial–organizational, tactile–perceptual, psychomotor, and non-verbal problem-solving and concept-formation skills, within a context of clear neuropsychological assets in some psycholinguistic skills such as rote verbal learning, regular phoneme–grapheme matching, amount of verbal output, and verbal classification. Children with NLD, a term coined by Myklebust (1975), experience their major academic learning difficulties in mechanical arithmetic, while exhibiting advanced levels of word-recognition and spelling. Both of these subtypes of children with LD have been the subject of much clinical and scientific inquiry in our laboratory (for basic research and reviews and some clinical examples, see Rourke, 1975, 1978, 1982, 1987, 1988a, 1988b, 1989, 1993; Rourke, Bakker, Fisk & Strang, 1983; Rourke & Del Dotto, 1994; Rourke & Finlayson, 1978; Rourke & Fisk, 1988, 1992; Rourke, Fisk & Strang, 1986; Rourke & Fuerst, 1991, 1992; Rourke & Strang, 1978, 1983; Strang & Rourke, 1983, 1985a, 1985b), and have been subjected to clinical, empirical and theoretical scrutiny by others (e.g. Bieliauskas, 1991; Fletcher, 1985; Sparrow, 1991; Torgeson, 1993; van der Vlugt, 1991; van der Vlugt & Satz, 1985).

Characteristics and dynamics of the NLD syndrome

The principal clinical manifestations (content) and dynamics of the NLD syndrome, that we identified through a process of intensive clinical examination, are as follows:

(1) Bilateral tactile–perceptual deficits, usually more marked on the left side of the body. Evidence of simple tactile imperception and suppression tends to subside with age, but problems in dealing with complex tactile input tend to persist.

(2) Bilateral psychomotor coordination deficiencies, often more marked on the left side of the body. Relatively simple motor skills, such as finger tapping and static steadiness, tend to normalize with advancing years. Complex psychomotor skills, especially when required within a novel framework, tend to worsen relative to age-based norms.

(3) Outstanding deficiencies in visual–spatial–organizational abilities. Simple visual discrimination, especially for material that is verbalizable, usually approaches normal levels with age. Complex visual–spatial–organizational skills, especially when required within a novel framework, tend to worsen relative to age-based norms.

(4) Extreme difficulty in adapting to novel and otherwise complex situations. An over-reliance on prosaic, rote (and, in consequence, inappropriate) behaviours in such situations. Capacity to deal with novel experiences usually remains poor, or even worsens, with advancing age.

(5) Marked deficits in non-verbal problem-solving, concept-formation, hypothesis-testing, and the capacity to benefit from positive and negative informational feedback in novel or otherwise complex situations. Included are significant difficulties in dealing with cause–effect relationships and marked deficiencies in the appreciation of incongruities (e.g. age-appropriate sensitivity to humour). Such deficiencies tend to persist, and even worsen, with advancing age.

(6) Very distorted sense of time. This is reflected in poor estimation of elapsed time during common activities, and poor estimation of time of day. (This deficit may not appear spontaneously; it usually requires a very direct attempt to elicit it.)

(7) Very well-developed rote verbal capacities, including extremely well-developed rote verbal memory skills. 'Memory' for complex verbal material is usually very poor, probably as a result of poor initial comprehension of such material.

(8) Much verbosity of a repetitive, straightforward, rote nature. Content disorders of language and very poor psycholinguistic pragmatics. Misspellings are almost exclusively of the phonetically accurate variety. Little or no speech prosody, except on an imitative basis. Excessive reliance upon language as a principal means for social relating, information gathering, and relief from anxiety.

(9) Outstanding relative deficiencies in mechanical arithmetic as compared to proficiencies in reading (word-recognition) and spelling. Comprehension of, as opposed to rote memory for, complex text may continue to be very poor with advancing age.

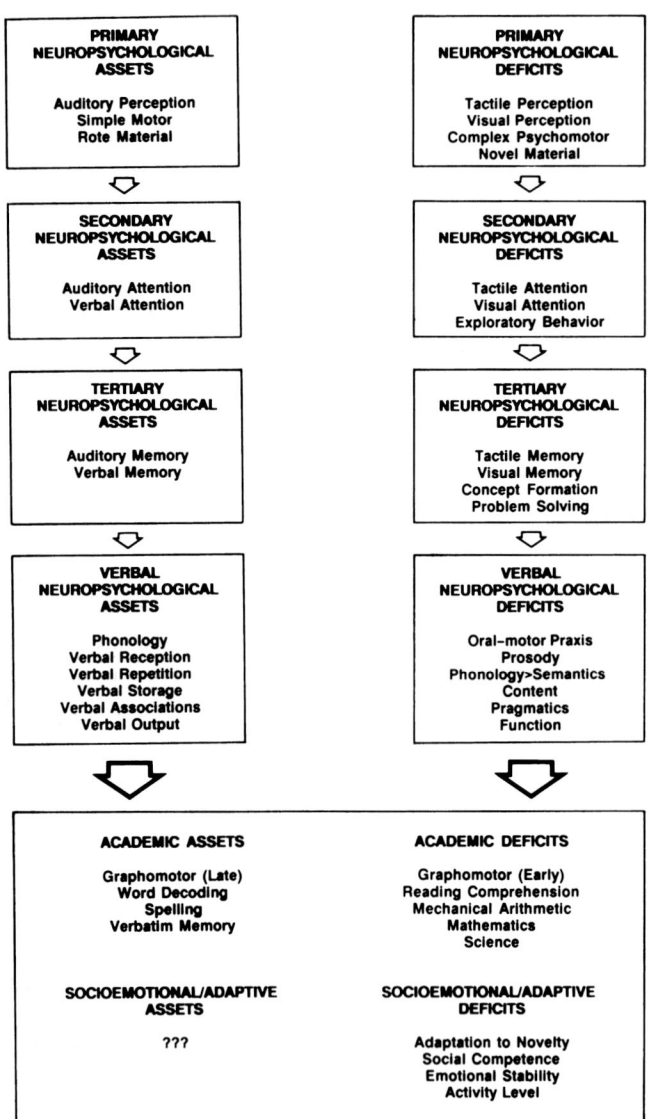

Fig. 2. Content and dynamics of the syndrome of non-verbal learning disabilities.

(10) Significant deficits in social perception, social judgement, and social interaction skills. During preschool and early school years, the child is often seen as 'hyperactive'. However, there is a marked tendency toward hypoactivity, often including social withdrawal and even social isolation, as age increases. There is considerable risk for the development of psychosocial disturbance, especially 'internalized' forms of psychopathology in older childhood and adolescence.

It is proposed in the model that the principal or primary dimensions of the NLD syndrome are deficits in visual–perceptual–organizational abilities, complex psychomotor skills, and tactile perception, in addition to difficulties in dealing with novelty. Primary assets include proficiency in most rote verbal and some simple motor and psychomotor skills (Rourke, 1989). These formulations were arrived at on the basis of clinical observations by ourselves and other practitioners. Confirmation of these dimensions as primary arises from the results of several studies (e.g. Casey *et al.*, 1991; Harnadek & Rourke, 1994). It should be emphasized that, in the Rourke (1989, 1995a) model, the patterns of academic and psychosocial assets and deficits experienced by individuals who exhibit NLD are viewed as the *direct* result of the interaction of the primary, secondary, tertiary, and linguistic neuropsychological assets and deficits that are outlined schematically in Fig. 2.

For example, considering the hypothesized 'deficit' stream, the primary neuropsychological deficits experienced by the child with NLD are seen as having to do with aspects of tactile and visual perception, complex psychomotor skills, and the capacity to deal adaptively with novel material. Such deficits would be expected to eventuate in disordered tactile and visual attention and stunted exploratory behaviour; in turn, problems in memory for material delivered through the tactile and visual modalities as well as deficits in concept-formation and problem-solving would be expected to ensue. This set of deficits would be expected to eventuate in the particular linguistic deficiencies outlined in Fig. 2 (see Rourke & Tsatsanis, 1995, for a fuller explanation of these linguistic deficits).

The academic and psychosocial/adaptive deficiencies listed are the expected sequelae of these neuropsychological deficits. It is especially important to note that this set of neuropsychological deficits is expected to lead, in a necessary way, to a particular configuration of problems in psychosocial/adaptive behaviour both within and without the academic situation (Rourke, 1988a, 1989, 1995a; Rourke & Fuerst, 1992). As suggested above, reference to Fig. 2 should be of some assistance in the understanding of our views regarding the content and dynamics of the NLD syndrome.

In a series of investigations (Casey *et al.*, 1991; Harnadek & Rourke, 1994; and see Rourke & Fuerst, 1991 for a summary of several studies), we have been able to demonstrate the concurrent and predictive validity of these formulations relating to the academic and psychosocial consequences of NLD. Also, it has been possible to demonstrate that particular patterns of academic assets and deficits are reliably related to particular patterns of psychosocial dysfunction across the age-span of interest (Fuerst & Rourke, 1995; Tsatsanis *et al.*, 1997). Thus, this investigative programme progressed from systematic clinical observations to the formulation of the NLD syndrome and dynamics and, eventually, to empirical tests of hypotheses deduced from the Rourke (1982, 1989, 1995a) models. Virtually all results of studies in our own and others' laboratories have been consistent with deductions derived from the neurodevelopmental models designed to encompass and explicate the NLD syndrome and its dynamics.

The white matter model

In addition to describing the content and dynamics of the NLD syndrome, a neuropsychological model to explain the syndrome's dynamics has been proposed (Rourke, 1987, 1988b, 1989; 1995a). The model involves an extension of the theoretical tenets of Goldberg & Costa (1981), some integration with Piagetian developmental theory, and some relationships to known age-related developmental changes in neuropsychological test performance.

For a full description of the syndrome and the 'white matter' model designed to account for it, the interested reader is referred to Rourke (1989, 1995a) and Tsatsanis & Rourke (1995a).

We have found that the NLD syndrome is manifest most clearly on a 'developmental' basis and that it persists into adulthood (Rourke & Fisk, 1992). However, it is also seen in the clinical presentation of persons suffering from a wide variety of types of neurological and neuroendocrine disease, disorder and dysfunction. These include significant tissue destruction within the right cerebral hemisphere (Rourke *et al.*, 1983) and some types of hydrocephalus (Fletcher *et al.*, 1995), callosal agenesis (Smith & Rourke, 1995), congenital hypothyroidism (Rovet, 1995) and other pathological processes that have as one of their results significant perturbation of neuronal white matter (long myelinated fibres). Other examples include persons with Williams syndrome (Anderson & Rourke, 1995; MacDonald & Roy, 1988; Udwin & Yule, 1991) and Asperger syndrome (Klin *et al.*, 1995), who exhibit virtually all of the assets and deficits of the NLD syndrome. A list and partial description of our current best estimates regarding these matters are contained in Table 1.

As may be clear from the foregoing, we are particularly interested to demonstrate the generalizability of the manifestations of the NLD syndrome. Indeed, we view the NLD syndrome as the final common pathway of a variety of neurological diseases and disorders (Rourke, 1987). As investigators pursue the clarification of the many dimensions of this question, the hierarchy originally proposed (Rourke, 1995a) has changed in some significant ways.

Table 1. Non-verbal learning disabilities: overview of manifestations in neurological disease, disorder and dysfunction

Level 1

Callosal dysgenesis (uncomplicated) (Rourke, 1987; Smith & Rourke, 1995)
Asperger syndrome (Klin *et al.*, 1995)
Velocardiofacial syndrome (Fuerst *et al.*, 1995; Golding-Kushner *et al.*, 1985; Moss *et al.*, 1998)
Williams syndrome (Anderson & Rourke, 1995; McDonald & Roy, 1988; Don *et al.*, 1999; Udwin & Yule, 1988)
de Lange syndrome (Tsatsanis & Rourke, 1995b)
Hydrocephalus (early; shunted) (Donders *et al.*, 1991; Fletcher *et al.*, 1992; Fletcher *et al.*, 1995; Rourke *et al.*, 1983, pp. 290–297)
Congenital hypothyroidism (Rovet, 1995a)
Significant damage or dysfunction of the right cerebral hemisphere (Rourke *et al.*, 1983, pp. 230–253)

Level 2

Turner syndrome (Rovet, 1995b) **(45, X: probably Level 1)**
Sotos syndrome (Dool *et al.*, 1995b)
Prophylactic treatment for all (long-term survivors) and other cancers (Buono *et al.*, 1998; Fletcher & Copeland, 1988; Picard & Rourke, 1995)
Metachromatic leukodystrophy (early in disease progression) (Dool *et al.*, 1995a; Shapiro *et al.*, 1992)
Fetal alcohol syndrome (high functioning) (Don & Rourke, 1995; Streissguth *et al.*, 1991)

Level 3

Multiple sclerosis (early to middle stages) (White & Krengel, 1995a)
Traumatic brain injury (diffuse white matter perturbations) (Ewing-Cobbs *et al.*, 1995; Fletcher & Levin, 1988)
Toxicant-induced encephalopathies (affecting white matter) (White & Krengel, 1995b)

Chapter 12 Non-verbal learning disabilities: development of the syndrome and the model

Some evidence of NLD

Children with HIV and white matter disease (Brouwers *et al.*, 1995)
Fragile X (high functioning) (Crowe & Hay, 1990)
Triple X syndrome (Ryan *et al.*, 1998)
Leukodystrophies other than metachromatic (early in disease)
Haemophilus influenzae **meningitis** (Taylor *et al.*, 1992)
Early-treated phenylketonuria (Faust *et al.*, 1986–87; Welsh *et al.*, 1990)
Intraventricular hemorrhage (early) (Landry *et al.*, 1993)
Congenital adrenal hyperplasia (Nass *et al.*, 1990)
Insulin dependent diabetes mellitus (very early onset) (Rovet, 1991)
Fahr's syndrome (Blackburn, 1996)

Ambiguous: neurofibromatosis (early to middle stages of disease progression) (Bawden *et al.*, 1996; Eliason, 1986; Nilsson & Bradford (1999); **Noonan Syndrome** (Troyer & Joschko, 1997)

Difficult to classify: cerebral palsies of perinatal origin

Similar, but basically different: Tourette syndrome (Brookshire *et al.*, 1994; Yeats & Bornstein, 1996); **Autism (high functioning)** (Klin *et al.*, 1995; Minshew *et al.*, 1994)

Notes:
(a) These forms of neurological disease, disorder and dysfunction are arranged in terms of a hierarchy. The levels within this hierarchy denote decreasing phenotypic similarity to the set of neuropsychological assets and deficits that constitute the manifestations of the NLD syndrome, as follows:

Level 1: **virtually all** of the NLD assets and deficits are manifest.

Level 2: a **considerable majority** of the NLD assets and deficits are evident.

Level 3: **many** of the NLD assets and deficits are manifested by a **significant subset** of children with these disorders.

(b) Prophylactic treatment, of course, is not a form of neurological disease. It is included at Level 2 because children who are long-term survivors of acute lymphoblastic leukaemia and who have received very high doses of whole brain cranial irradiation and some other types of therapies frequently exhibit a considerable majority of the NLD assets and deficits.

(c) The category labelled 'suggestive' contains a number of diseases where the literature is highly suggestive of patterns of NLD assets and deficits emergent in a significant subset of children so afflicted. These diseases are being examined from the perspective of the NLD/white matter model in the future.

(d) Many children with cerebral palsy of perinatal origin exhibit a considerable majority of the NLD assets and deficits. However, because of the wide variety of aetiologies and manifestations considered under this rubric, the classification by level of NLD manifestations is rendered problematic.

(e) Tourette syndrome (TS) is one example of a neurological disorder wherein several of the NLD manifestations are evident. However, there are many basic differences that suggest strongly that TS is not a syndrome that should be considered within the group of neurological disorders that can be characterized in terms of the NLD spectrum (Brookshire *et al.*, 1994). A similar state of affairs obtains with respect to 'high functioning' autism (Klin *et al.*, 1995).

(f) It is very probable that this hierarchy will change somewhat as more is known about the neuropsychological manifestations of the diseases in question.

(g) It is likely that other forms of neurological disease, disorder, and dysfunction will be added to this hierarchy.

(h) It would appear highly probable that advances in neuroimaging of white matter functioning, neuropathological findings regarding white matter perturbations, and other advances in the specification of the developmental and functional neuroanatomy of myelination will throw considerable light upon the underpinnings of this NLD hierarchy.

Treatment

A treatment programme for children with NLD that has been applied with some success is outlined in Rourke (1989) and Rourke (1995b). We have taken considerable pains to relate the elements of this programme to the content and dynamics of the NLD syndrome. In addition, we have suggested explicit strategies and interventions whose efficacy can be tested by empirical means. It is anticipated that the continuation of investigations and applications of the programme in various centres (e.g. Cermak & Murray, 1992; Cracco & Thierry, 1993; Foss, 1991; Williams et al., 1992), including our own (e.g. Ozols & Rourke, 1991; Rourke & Tsatsanis, 1995), will yield important information with respect to its efficacy and, in turn, lead to refinements of it.

Conclusions

We have addressed the issue of 'right hemisphere' disorders and their consequences from a perspective that has been developed over a number of years and through a large number of investigations in our own and others' laboratories. Our conclusions with respect to the syndrome of NLD are quite clear: the syndrome is apparent in many indidividuals who have significant perturbations of right hemisphere systems; thus, significant dysfunction within the right cerebral hemisphere is seen as a *sufficient* condition for the appearance of the NLD syndrome. The syndrome is also apparent in many individuals with significant perturbations of long myelinated fibres (white matter disease) in many, if not most, regions of the brain; thus, significant perturbations of white matter appear to be *necessary* to 'produce' the NLD syndrome. It remains for further research to delineate whether and to what extent these inferences stand up to scientific scrutiny.

References

Anderson, P. & Rourke, B.P. (1995): Williams syndrome. In: *Syndrome of nonverbal learning disabilities: neurodevelopmental manifestations*, ed. B.P. Rourke, pp. 138–170. New York: Guilford Press.

Bawden, H., Dooley, J., Buckley, D., Camfield, P., Gordon, K., Riding, M. & Llewellyn, G. (1996): MRI and nonverbal cognitive deficits in children with neurofibromatosis 1. *J Clin. Exp. Neuropsychol.* **18**, 784–792.

Bieliauskas, L.A. (1991): Case studies of adults with nonverbal learning disabilities. In: *Neuropsychological validation of learning disability subtypes*, ed. B.P. Rourke, pp. 370–376. New York: Guilford Press.

Blackburn, L.B. (1996): Neurodevelopmental course in pediatric onset progressive calcification of the basal ganglion: a case report. *Arch. Clin. Neuropsychol.* **11**, 369–370

Brookshire, B., Butler, I.J., Ewing-Cobbs, L. & Fletcher, J.M. (1994): Neuropsychological characteristics of children with Tourette syndrome: evidence for a nonverbal learning disability? *J. Clin. Exp. Neuropsychol.* **16**, 289–302.

Brouwers, P., van der Vlugt, H., Moss, H., Wolters, P. & Pizzo, P. (1995): White matter changes on CT brain scan are associated with neurobehavioral dysfunction in children with symptomatic HIV disease. *Child Neuropsychol.* **1**, 93–105.

Buono, L.A., Morris, M. K., Morris, R.D., Krawiecki, N., Norris, F.H., Foster, M.A. & Copeland, D.R. (1998): Evidence for the syndrome of Nonverbal Learning Disabilities in children with brain tumors. *Child Neuropsychol.* **4**, 144–157.

Casey, J.E., Rourke, B.P. & Picard, E.M. (1991): Syndrome of nonverbal learning disabilities: age differences in neuropsychological, academic, and socioemotional functioning. *Dev. Psychopathol.* **3**, 329–345.

Cermak, S.A. & Murray, E. (1992): Nonverbal learning disabilities in the adult framed in the model of human occupation. In: *Cognitive rehabilitation: models for intervention in occupational therapy,* ed. N. Katz, pp. 258–291. Boston: Andover Medical.

Cracco, J. & Thierry, E. (1993): Neuropsychological assessment and treatment plan for a girl with nonverbal learning disabilities: a case study. *Acta Ergotherapeutica Belgica* **5,** 103–111.

Crowe, S.F. & Hay, D.A. (1990): Neuropsychological dimensions of the fragile X syndrome: support for a non-dominant hemisphere dysfunction hypothesis. *Neuropsychologia* **28,** 9–16.

DeLuca, J.W. (1991): Case studies of adolescents with nonverbal learning disabilities. In: *Neuropsychological validation of learning disability subtypes,* ed. B.P. Rourke, pp. 356–369. New York: Guilford Press.

Don, A. & Rourke, B.P. (1995): Fetal alcohol syndrome. In: *Syndrome of nonverbal learning disabilities: neurodevelopmental manifestations,* ed. B.P. Rourke, pp. 372–406. New York: Guilford Press.

Don, A., Schellenberg, G. & Rourke, B.P. (1999): Auditory pattern perception in children with Williams syndrome. *Child Neuropsychol.* **5.**

Donders, J.,Rourke, B.P. & Canady, A.I. (1991): Neuropsychological functioning of hydrocephalic children. *J. Clin. Exp. Neuropsychol.* **13,** 607–613.

Dool, C.B., Fuerst, K.B. & Rourke, B.P. (1995a): Metachromatic leukodystrophy. In: *Syndrome of nonverbal learning disabilities: neurodevelopmental manifestations,* ed. B.P. Rourke, pp. 331–350. New York: Guilford Press.

Dool, C.B., Fuerst, K.B. & Rourke, B.P. (1995b): Sotos syndrome. In: *Syndrome of nonverbal learning disabilities: neurodevelopmental manifestations,* ed. B.P. Rourke. New York: Guilford Press.

Eliason, M.J. (1986): Neurofibromatosis: implications for learning and behavior. *J. Dev. Behav. Pediatr.* **7,** 175–179.

Ewing-Cobbs, L., Fletcher, J. M. & Levin, H.S. (1995): Traumatic brain injury. In: *Syndrome of nonverbal learning disabilities: neurodevelopmental manifestations,* ed. B.P. Rourke, pp. 433–459. New York: Guilford Press.

Faust, D., Libon, D. & Pueschel, S. (1986–87): Neuropsychological functioning in treated phenylketonuria. *Int. J. Psychiatr. Med.* **16,** 169–177.

Fletcher, J.M. (1985): External validation of learning disability typologies. In: *Neuropsychology of learning disabilities: essentials of subtype analysis,* ed. B.P. Rourke, pp. 187–211. New York: Guilford Press.

Fletcher, J.M. & Copeland, D.R. (1988): Neurobehavioral effects of central nervous system prophylactic treatment of cancer in children. *J. Clin. Exp. Neuropsychol.* **10,** 495–537.

Fletcher, J.M. & Levin, H. (1988): Neurobehavioral effects of brain injury in children. In: *Handbook of pediatric psychology,* ed. D.K. Routh, pp. 258–295. New York: Guilford Press.

Fletcher, J.M., Bohan, T.P., Brandt, M.E., Brookshire, B.L., Beaver, S.R., Francis, D.J., Davidson, K.C., Thompson, N.M. & Milner, M.E. (1992): Cerebral white matter and cognition in hydrocephalic children. *Arch. Neurol.* **49,** 818–825.

Fletcher, J.M., Francis, D.J., Thompson, N.M., Brookshire, B.L., Bohan, T.P., Landry, S.H., Davidson, K.C. & Miner, M.E. (1992): Verbal and nonverbal skill discrepancies in hydrocephalic children. *J. Clin. Exp. Neuropsychol.* **14,** 593–609.

Fletcher, J.M., Brookshire, B.L., Bohan, T.P., Brandt, M. & Davidson, K. (1995): Early hydrocephalus. In: *Syndrome of nonverbal learning disabilities: neurodevelopmental manifestations,* ed. B.P. Rourke, pp. 206–238. New York: Guilford Press.

Foss, J.M. (1991): Nonverbal learning disabilities and remedial interventions. *Ann. Dyslexia* **41,** 128–140.

Fuerst, D.R. & Rourke, B.P. (1995): Psychosocial functioning of children with learning disabilities at three age levels. *Child Neuropsychol.* **1,** 38–55.

Fuerst, K.B., Dool, C.B. & Rourke, B.P. (1995): Velocardiofacial syndrome. In: *Syndrome of nonverbal learning disabilities: neurodevelopmental manifestations,* ed. B.P. Rourke, pp. 119–137. New York: Guilford Press.

Golding-Kushner, K.J., Weller, G. & Shprintzen, R.J. (1985): Velo-cardio-facial syndrome: language and psychological profiles. *J. Craniofacial Gen. Dev. Biol.* **5**, 259–266.

Harnadek, M.C.S. & Rourke, B.P. (1994): Principal identifying features of the syndrome of nonverbal learning disabilities in children. *J. Learning Disabilities* **27**, 144–154.

Klin, A., Sparrow, S.S., Volkmar, F., Cicchetti, D.V. & Rourke, B.P. (1995): Asperger syndrome. In: *Syndrome of nonverbal learning disabilities: neurodevelopmental manifestations,* ed. B.P. Rourke, pp. 93–118. New York: Guilford Press.

Klin, A., Volkmar, F.R., Sparrow, S.S., Cicchetti, D.V. & Rourke, B.P. (1995): Validity and neuropsychological characterization of Asperger sundrome: Convergence with Nonverbal Learning Disabilities syndrome. *J. Child Psychol. Psychiatr.* **36**, 1127–1140.

Landry, S.H., Fletcher, J.M. & Denson, S.E. (1993): Longitudinal outcome for low birth weight infants: effects of intraventricular hemorrhage and bronchopulmonary dysplasia. *J. Clin. Exp. Neuropsychol.* **15**, 205–218.

MacDonald, G.W. & Roy, D.L. (1988): Williams syndrome: a neuropsychological profile. *J. Clin. Exp. Neuropsychol.* **10**, 125–131.

Minshew, N.J., Goldstein, G., Taylor, H.G. & Siegel, D.J. (1994): Academic achievement in high functioning autistic individuals. *J. Clin. Exp. Neuropsychol.* **16**, 671–680.

Moss, E.M., Wang, P.P., McGinn, D.M., Keating, T.B., Sugama, S., Driscott, D.A., Emanual, B.S., Batshaw, M.L. & Zackai, E.H. (1998): Genetic insights into nonverbal learning disabilities: the cognitive and adaptive profiles of patients with a chromosome 22q11.2 microdeletion. Paper presented at the meeting of the American Psychological Association, San Francisco.

Myklebust, H.R. (1975): Nonverbal learning disabilities: Assessment and intervention. In: *Progress in learning disabilities,* vol. 3, ed. H.R. Myklebust, pp. 85–121. New York: Grune & Stratton.

Nass, R. Speiser, P., Heier, L., Haimes, A. & New, M. (1990): White matter abnormalities in congenital adrenal hyperplasia. *Ann. Neurol.* **28**, 470.

Nilsson, D.E. & Bradford, L.W. (1999): Neurofibromatosis. In: *Handbook of neurodevelopmental and genetic disorders in children*, eds. S. Goldstein & C.R. Reynolds, pp. 350–367. New York: Guilford Press.

Ozols, E.J. & Rourke, B.P. (1991): Classification of young learning-disabled children according to patterns of academic achievement: validity studies. In: *Neuropsychological validation of learning disability subtypes,* ed. B.P. Rourke, pp. 97–123. New York: Guilford Press.

Picard, E.M. & Rourke, B.P. (1995): Neuropsychological consequences of prophylactic treatment for acute lymphocytic leukaemia. In: *Syndrome of nonverbal learning disabilities: neurodevelopmental manifestations*, ed. B.P. Rourke, pp. 282–330. New York: Guilford Press.

Rourke, B.P. (1975): Brain-behavior relationships in children with learning disabilities. *Am. Psychol.* **30**, 911–920.

Rourke, B.P. (1978): Reading, spelling, arithmetic disabilities: a neuropsychologic perspective. In: *Progress in learning disabilities,* ed. H.R. Myklebust, vol. 4, pp. 97–120. New York: Grune & Stratton.

Rourke, B.P. (1982): Central processing deficiencies in children: toward a developmental neuropsychological model. *J. Clin. Neuropsychol.* **4**, 1–18.

Rourke, B.P. (1987): Syndrome of nonverbal learning disabilities: the final common pathway of white-matter disease/dysfunction? *Clin. Neuropsychol.* **1**, 209–234.

Rourke, B.P. (1988a): Socioemotional disturbances of learning disabled children. *J. Consulting Clin. Psychol.* **56**, 801–810.

Rourke, B.P. (1988b): The syndrome of nonverbal learning disabilities: developmental manifestations in neurological disease, disorder, and dysfunction. *Clin. Neuropsychol.* **2**, 293–330.

Rourke, B.P. (1989): *Nonverbal learning disabilities: the syndrome and the model.* New York: Guilford Press.

Rourke, B.P. (1991): *Neuropsychological validation of learning disability subtypes.* New York: Guilford Press.

Rourke, B.P. (1993): Arithmetic disabilities, specific and otherwise: a neuropsychological perspective. *J. Learning Disabilities* **26,** 214–226.

Rourke, B.P. (1995a): *Syndrome of nonverbal learning disabilities: neurodevelopmental manifestations.* New York: Guilford Press.

Rourke, B.P. (1995b): Treatment program for children and adolescents with NLD. In: *Syndrome of nonverbal learning disabilities: neurodevelopmental manifestations,* ed. B.P. Rourke, pp. 497–508. New York: Guilford Press.

Rourke, B.P., Bakker, D.J., Fisk, J.L. & Strang, J.D. (1983): *Child neuropsychology: an introduction to theory, research, and clinical practice.* New York: Guilford Press.

Rourke, B.P. & Finlayson, M.A.J. (1978): Neuropsychological significance of variations in patterns of academic performance: verbal and visual–spatial abilities. *J. Abnormal Child Psychol.* **6,** 121–133.

Rourke, B.P. & Fisk, J.L. (1992): Adult presentations of learning disabilities. In: *Clinical syndromes in adult neuropsychology: the practitioner's handbook,* ed. R.F. White, pp. 451–473. Amsterdam: Elsevier.

Rourke, B.P. & Fuerst, D.R. (1991): *Learning disabilities and psychosocial functioning.* New York: Guilford Press.

Rourke, B.P. & Fuerst, D.R. (1992): Psychosocial dimensions of learning disability subtypes: neuropsychological studies in the Windsor Laboratory. *Sch. Psychol. Rev.* **21,** 360–373.

Rourke, B.P. & Del Dotto, J.E. (1994): *Learning disabilities: A neuropsychological perspective.* Thousand Oaks, CA: Sage.

Rourke, B.P. & Fisk, J.L. (1988): Subtypes of learning-disabled children: Implications for a neurodevelopmental model of differential hemispheric processing. In: *Brain lateralization in children: Developmental implications,* eds. D.L. Molfese & S.J. Segalowitz, pp. 547–565. New York: Guilford Press.

Rourke, B.P. & Strang, J.D. (1978): Neuropsychological significance of variations in patterns of academic performance: motor, psychomotor, and tactile–perceptual abilities. *J. Pediatr. Psychol.* **3,** 62–66.

Rourke, B.P. & Strang, J.D. (1983): Subtypes of reading and arithmetical disabilities: a neuropsychological analysis. In: *Developmental neuropsychiatry,* ed. M. Rutter, pp. 473–488. New York: Guilford Press.

Rourke, B.P. & Tsatsanis, K.D. (1995): Memory disturbances of children with learning disabilities: a neuropsychological analysis of two academic achievement subtypes. In: *Handbook of memory disorders,* eds. A.D. Baddeley, B.A. Wilson & F.N. Watts, pp. 501–531. London: Wiley & Sons.

Rourke, B.P., Fisk, J.L. & Strang, J.D. (1986): *Neuropsychological assessment of children: A treatment-oriented approach.* New York: Guilford Press.

Rovet, J.F. (1991): Learning disabilities profiles in four endocrine disorders. *J. Clin. Exp. Neuropsychol.* **13,** 58–59.

Rovet, J.F. (1995a): Congenital hypothyroidism. In: *Syndrome of nonverbal learning disabilities: neurodevelopmental manifestations,* ed. B.P. Rourke, pp. 255–281. New York: Guilford Press.

Rovet, J.F. (1995b): Turner syndrome. In: *Syndrome of nonverbal learning disabilities: Neurodevelopmental manifestations,* ed. B.P. Rourke, pp. 351–371.

Ryan, T.V., Crews, Jr., W.D., Cowan, L., Goering, A.M. & Barth, J.T. (1998): A case of triple X syndrome manifesting with the syndrome of nonverbal learning disabilities. *Child Neuropsychol.* **4,** 225–232.

Shapiro, E.G., Lipton, M.E. & Krivit, W. (1992): White matter dysfunction and its neuropsychological correlates: a longitudinal study of a case of metachromatic leukodystrophy treated with bone marrow transplant. *J. Clin. Exp. Neuropsychol.* **14,** 610–624.

Smith, L.A. & Rourke, B.P. (1995): Callosal agenesis. In *Syndrome of nonverbal learning disabilities: neurodevelopmental manifestations,* ed. B.P. Rourke, pp. 45–92. New York: Guilford Press.

Sparrow, S.S. (1991): Case studies of children with nonverbal learning disabilities. In: *Neuropsychological validation of learning disability subtypes,* ed. B.P. Rourke, pp. 349–355. New York: Guilford Press.

Strang, J.D. & Rourke, B.P. (1983): Concept-formation/non-verbal reasoning abilities of children who exhibit specific academic problems with arithmetic. *J. Clin. Child Psychol.* **12,** 33–39.

Strang, J.D. & Rourke, B.P. (1985a): Adaptive behavior of children with specific arithmetic disabilities and associated neuropsychological abilities and deficits. In: *Neuropsychology of learning disabilities: essentials of subtype analysis,* ed. B.P. Rourke, pp. 302–328. New York: Guilford Press.

Strang, J.D. & Rourke, B.P. (1985b): Arithmetic disability subtypes: the neuropsychological significance of specific arithmetical impairment in childhood. In: *Neuropsychology of learning disabilities: essentials of subtype analysis,* ed. B.P. Rourke, pp. 167–183. New York: Guilford Press.

Streissguth, A.P., Aase, J.M., Clarren, S.K., Randels, S.P., LaDue, R.A. & Smith, D.F. (1991): Fetal alcohol syndrome in adolescents and adults. *J. Am. Med. Assoc.* **265,** 1961–1967.

Taylor, H.G., Schatschneider, C. & Rich, D. (1992): Sequelae of *Haemophilus influenzae* meningitis: implications for the study of brain disease and development. In: *Advances in child neuropsychology,* eds. M.G. Tramontana & S.R. Hooper, vol. 1, pp. 50–108. New York: Springer-Verlag.

Torgeson, J.K. (1993): Variations on theory in learning disabilities. In: *Better understanding learning disabilities: new views from research and their implications for education and public policies,* eds. G.R. Lyon, D.B. Gray, J.F. Kavanagh & N.A. Krasnegor, pp. 153–170. Baltimore, MD: Paul H. Brookes.

Troyer, A.K. & Joschko, M. (1997): Cognitive characteristics associated with Noonan Syndrome: two case reports. *Child Neuropsychol.* **3,** 199–205.

Tsatsanis, K.D. & Rourke, B.P. (1995a): Conclusions and future directions. In: *Syndrome of nonverbal learning disabilities: neurodevelopmental manifestations,* ed. B.P. Rourke, pp. 476–496. New York: Guilford Press.

Tsatsanis, K.D. & Rourke, B.P. (1995b): de Lange syndrome. In: *Syndrome of nonverbal learning disabilities: neurodevelopmental manifestations,* ed. B.P. Rourke, pp. 171–205. New York: Guilford Press.

Tsatsanis, K.D., Fuerst, D.R. & Rourke, B.P. (1997): Psychosocial dimensions of learning disabilities: External validation and relationship with age and academic functioning. *J. Learning Disabil.* **30,** 490–502.

Udwin, O. & Yule, W. (1991): A cognitive and behavioral phenotype in Williams syndrome. *J. Clin. Exp. Neuropsychol.* **13,** 232–244.

Udwin, O. & Yule, W. (1988): *Infantile hypercalcaemia and Williams syndrome: guidelines for parents.* Essex, United Kingdom: Infantile Hypercalcaemia Foundation.

van der Vlugt, H. (1991): Neuropsychological validation studies of learning disability subtypes: Verbal, visual–spatial, and psychomotor abilities. In: *Neuropsychological validation of learning disability subtypes,* ed. B.P. Rourke, pp. 140–159. New York: Guilford Press.

van der Vlugt, H. & Satz, P. (1985): Subgroups and subtypes of learning-disabled and normal children: A cross-cultural replication. In: *Neuropsychology of learning disabilities: Essentials of subtype analysis,* ed. B.P Rourke, pp. 212–227. New York: Guilford Press.

Welsh, M.C., Pennington, B.F., Rouse, B. & McCabe, E.R.B. (1990): Neuropsychology of early-treated phenylketonuria: specific executive function deficits. *Child Dev.* **61,** 1697–1713.

White, R.F. & Krengel, M. (1995a): Multiple sclerosis. In: *Syndrome of nonverbal learning disabilities: neurodevelopmental manifestations,* ed. B.P. Rourke. New York: Guilford Press.

White, R.F. & Krengel, M. (1995b): Toxicant-induced encephalopathy. In: *Syndrome of nonverbal learning disabilities: neurodevelopmental manifestations,* ed. B.P. Rourke, pp. 460–475. New York: Guilford Press.

Williams, J.K., Richman, L. & Yarbrough, D. (1992): Comparison of visual spatial performance strategy training in children with Turner syndrome and learning disabilities. *J. Learning Disabilities* **25,** 658–664.

Yeates, K.O. & Bornstein, R.A. (1996): Psychosocial correlates of learning disability subtypes in children with Tourette's syndrome. *Child Neuropsychol.* **2,** 193–203.

Chapter 13

Congenital lesions of cerebellum

Francesco Guzzetta, Eugenio Mercuri, Maria Spanò and
Maria Flavia Frisone

Neuropsichiatria Infantile, Università Cattolica del Sacro Cuore, Policlinico Gemelli, Largo Gemelli 8, 00168 Rome, Italy

Summary

A short review of developmental disorders of cerebellum is presented. Special emphasis has been given to a form of congenital atrophy, and the possible relationship between cerebellar defects and cognitive development is also stressed.

Embryological notes

After 3 weeks gestation the first growth of the rostral segment of the neural tube, which is anchored at two fixed points (bucco-pharingeal membrane and cervical somites), produces two main flexures, the cephalic and the cervical. During the fifth week the pontine flexure will form between. Cellular multiplication at the alar plate is associated with differentiation of various groups of cells (neuroblasts) and their dorsal and medial migration from the rombic lips will form the cerebellum. The first type of migrating cells will be the Purkjnie cells, followed by stellar and basket cells, and eventually by granular cells that in a first stage will be located at the external cortical layer. Afterwards, guided by the Bergman glia, granular cells will migrate into the deepest layer of the cerebellar cortex.

The migration process will be completed only several months after birth (9–12 m). The cellular group located at the extreme lateral corner of the rombic lips will rostrally determine the flocculo-nodular lobe of the cerebellum and caudally the vestibular nuclei in the medulla (archicerebellum).

The first transverse fissura to appear (45th day) is the fissura posterolateralis that separates the flocculo-nodular lobe from the rest of the cerebellum, followed by the fissura prima (70th day), which divides the anterior from the posterior part. The other fissurae will subsequently form to divide the cerebellar folia. The first part to be accomplished is the vermis.

Cerebellum phylogenesis as well as ontogenesis defines three different functional parts of the cerebellum:

archicerebellum (or vestibulo-cerebellum) located in the flocculo-nodular lobe;

paleocerebellum (or spinocerebellum) located in the vermis and the intermediate parts;

neocerebellum (pontocerebellum or cerebro-cerebellum) formed by the rest of the cerebellar hemispheres.

Nosography of the cerebellar malformations

The nosography of the cerebellar malformations is generally embryologically based. Two main groups, paleo and neocerebellar malformations, can be identified according to the timing of the developmental error.

Paleocerebellar malformations are typically characterized by a vermian agenesia or dysgenesia. Cystic forms are frequent and include some syndromes (Dandy Walker, Dandy Walker variant) in which malformations originate from a developmental lesion of the anterior membraneous area. Other cystic forms, such as cisterna hypermagna and the pocket of Blake, are malformations of the posterior membranous area.

Non-cystic forms include very rare cases of vermis agenesia like rombencenphalosynapsis or tecto-cerebellar dysraphia.

Paleocerebellar malformations are very often genetic in origin and frequently part of more pervasive and peculiar malformative syndromes (Joubert, Klippel-Feil, de Lange etc.). Clinical signs associated with paleocerebellar malformations are severe motor impairment and mental retardation, and other signs of supratentorial lesions (seizures, visual impairment, etc.).

Neocerebellar malformations include more or less extensive agenesia of the hemispheres, often caused by a destructive vascular accident, and the less severe but more diffuse forms of cortical dysgenesia, such as cerebellar hypoplasia or hypotrophia, whose origin is more heterogeneous.

An acquired case is that of the cerebellar hemihypotrophy found contralaterally to congenital extensive infarction of a cerebral hemisphere due to a transneuronal degeneration of the cerebellar cortex.

The clinical picture associated with neocerebellar malformations consists of a mild cerebellar syndrome not associated with other signs of supratentorial involvement.

Role of the cerebellum in motor and cognitive development

In this paper we will briefly review some aspects of the cerebellar pathophysiology in relation to movement. We will also review the possible role of the cerebellum in cognitive development, reporting our experience in a population of children with isolated congenital cerebellar malformation.

The role of the cerebellum in the regulation of muscular activity is well known. Although cerebellar signs cannot be always easily related to specific lesions of definite parts of the cerebellum, there are at least two main categories of neurological signs which have been observed in isolation in congenital cerebellar pathology (De Negri et al., 1987). The first one consists of titubation and difficulty in maintaining equilibrium and is generally recorded as truncal ataxia. The other dissimulates, in an apparently variegated symptomatology (hypotonia, intentional tremor, dysmetria/hypermetria, nystagmus, dysarthria) a possibly unique mechanism of asynergia, defined by Holmes (1939) as a 'decomposition of movement'.

These clinical patterns are usually associated with two specific patterns of congenital lesions: the early pathology especially involving the vermian region accounts for the dysequilibrium syndrome (Hagberg et al., 1972) while in neocerebellar lesions asynergia is mostly commonly found.

Beside the regulation of muscular activity, there is growing evidence that cerebellum is involved in the mechanisms of motor skill learning, since Marr (1969) and Albus (1971) suggested the well-known model of cerebellar plasticity in adapting behaviour to motor tasks, based on the double inputs to the Purkinje cells (climbing fibres originating from the inferior olive and mossy fibres originating from the pontine nuclei). The first one provides 'teaching' information concerning changes in needs of muscular activity, whilst the second kind of inputs produces the 'learning' of new associations relating to the movement adaptation. In Pavlovian terms, stimulation of climbing fibres works as an unconditioned teaching stimulus, whereas activation of mossy fibres as a conditioned learning stimulus (Lavonde et al., 1987). Electrophysiological evidence of motor learning was provided by Gilbert & Thach (1977). Recording EEG, they were able to show a critical increase of complex spike activity during the process of motor learning in new movement situations, expressing the climbing fibre inputs: when the new task is learned, the complex spike activity goes down to the usual rate.

A disturbed motor learning was shown in cerebellar pathology as a lack of plasticity in motor adaptation to visual environment when altered by wearing distorting prisms (Gauthier et al., 1979; Weiner et al., 1983). Recently, Sanes et al. (1990) showed this kind of cerebellar dysfunction in congenital cerebellar atrophy or in cerebellar atrophy associated with atrophy of the brain stem (olivo-ponto-cerebellar atrophy: OPCA).

Increasing attention has been devoted in the last years to the possible role of the cerebellum in cognitive function. There are at least four kinds of findings suggesting that the integrity of the cerebellum is necessary for normal cognitive development:

(1) developmental cognitive problems in patients with cerebellar diseases without supratentorial involvement;

(2) results of functional studies of the human cerebellum with neuroimaging techniques (SPECT, PET, functional MRI) in subjects performing neuropsychological tasks;

(3) findings of functional cerebello-cerebral connections through studies of crossed cerebellar diaschisis;

(4) anatomical evidence for cerebellar involvement in cognitive function showed by retrograde transneuronal transport of viruses (HSV1).

Several neuropsychological studies have reported definite cognitive deficits in patients with either cerebellar disease, such as Friedreich ataxia (Hart et al., 1986), or atrophy of cerebellar cortex (Grafman et al., 1992), as well as in cases with acquired pathology (phenytoin intoxication: Botez et al., 1985) showing the involvement of cognition. Using the Tower of Hanoi in subjects with cortical cerebellar atrophy, Grafman et al. (1992) demonstrated evidence of a frontal-like syndrome (concerning cognitive planning). Cognitive planning can be considered as a mental representation of the motor process consisting of a coherent series of movements or motor sequences (Ito, 1990). One can imagine that, as shown in the execution of movements, there is a cerebellar competence inside the cerebello-frontal axis concerning function of temporal on-line integration of events. Beside the cognitive planning deficit (cerebello-frontal loop), a visuo-spatial organization fault linked to the cerebello-parietal loop and a decrease of the speed of information processing (Botez, 1992) were shown in cerebellar patients. A deficit of mental performances related to concrete thought completes the cognitive profile of the patients with isolated cerebellar diseases.

Neuropsychological findings in cerebellar pathology were confirmed by functional neuroimaging examinations. PET and SPECT studies showed a metabolic activation in cerebellar hemispheres during mental activity such as language processing (Petersen et al., 1989) or mental counting (Ryding et al., 1993); this activation was topographically and quantitatively differentiated from the activation due to simple motor activity.

To prove the role of the cerebellar output in cognitive functions, Kim et al. (1994) studied the involvement of the dentate nucleus. The examination with functional MRI of subjects during attempts to solve a pegboard puzzle showed a significantly greater activation of the dentate nucleus than when simple movements of pegs were being performed.

Neuropathological studies have supplied further evidence of the cerebro-cerebellar pathways which might be involved in cognitive functioning. First of all, the phenomenon of the so-called crossed cerebellar diaschisis, i.e. the metabolic depression shown by PET studies (Baron et al., 1980; Meneghetti et al., 1984; Feeney & Baron, 1986; Pantano et al., 1986) in the cerebellar hemisphere contralateral to a cerebral lesion (e.g. a stroke). If persistent, it can become a real cerebellar atrophy due to transneuronal degeneration (cortico-ponto-cerebellar pathways), such as we can observe in some cases of congenital infarction due to occlusion of the silvian artery. More recently, Botez et al. (1991) have shown the reversed phenomenon of cerebello-cerebral diaschisis caused by a cerebellar infarction or even in congenital cerebellar pathology such as Friedreich ataxia or olivo-ponto-cerebellar atrophy: two pathways seem involved, the cerebello-thalamo-cortical (frontal and parietal) loop and a dopaminergic pathway through the basal ganglia.

Finally, there is anatomical evidence for specific cerebellar pathways of cognitive functions showed by experimental studies with retrograde transneuronal transport of herpes simplex type 1 (HSV1). Middleton & Strick (1994) have proved a connection between the frontal pre-motor area and restricted regions of the nucleus dentatus, a loop related to higher cognitive functions that are not the same regions of the nucleus connected with the motor area.

Clinical study: the case of congenital cerebellar atrophy

Although experimental and pathological studies have supplied interesting points supporting the role of the cerebellum in cognitive development, few studies have been able to show a correlation between cerebellar lesions proven with imaging, and cognitive deficits in children. This is mainly due to the fact that, unlike adult stroke, isolated cerebellar lesions, without any involvement of the supratentorial structure, are very rare in childhood. Furthermore, mental retardation is often so severe as to make it impossible to delineate a cerebellar profile of the cognitive deficit.

We present a study concerning 10 patients affected with a chronic, non-progressive, congenital, cerebellar atrophy, which for its pathological identity we think can be considered as a model for the study of the role of the cerebellum in cognitive development.

These cases we partially reported (Guzzetta et al., 1993) presented with:

(1) mild cerebellar neurological syndrome;

(2) mild mental retardation;

(3) sporadic or familial occurrence, consistent with a pattern of autosomal recessive inheritance;

(4) no metabolic markers and no chemical and neuroimaging evidence of progression;

(5) diffuse cerebellar cortical atrophy with a slight enlargement of the fourth ventricle;

(6) no signs of associated supratentorial changes.

On the basis of similarity with other autoptically studied cases (Norman, 1940; Jervis, 1950), our patients can be supposed to be affected with a cortical dysplasia due to early degeneration and/or necrosis of migrating granule cells; this is why we prefer to use the denomination of cerebellar atrophy rather than hypoplasia.

The isolated involvement of the cerebellar cortex at an early stage of development allowed us to study the cognition profile and to relate it with the congenital cerebellar pathology.

Neuropsychological assessments paid special attention to visuo-spatial organization, information processing speed, and motor learning.

All the children in our study group showed global cognitive impairment on the Wechsler Intelligence scales. However, performance was significantly more affected than language. More specifically, perceptual and motor organizations were the most affected, with the lowest scores in the items that assessed motor activity guided by visual organization (arithmetic, mazes, object assembly, digit symbol, block design).

The speed of information processing, evaluated on a movement/reaction time test, was also very low, even by comparison with a mentally retarded control group, matched for age and IQ. Moreover, the adaptive process following the mirror-reversed test of Corsi was impaired, suggesting a dysfunction in motor learning. Even though this study should be validated by tests assessing planning skills, these results provide some points in favour of a role of the cerebellum in cognitive development.

As a result, many interesting clinical questions arise, such as:

(1) how could the lack of the adaptive process in motor learning impair the mechanism of motor scheme integration on which the beginning of mental development depends, according to Piaget's theory?

(2) to what extent is it possible to use neuropsychological assessment as a diagnostic and prognostic tool in congenital cerebellar diseases?

(3) which kind of suggestion can be drawn from this kind of cerebellar pathology for the motor and cognitive development?

References

Albus, J.S. (1971): A theory of cerebellar function. *Math. Biosci.* **10**, 25–61.

Baron, J.C., Bousser, M.G., Comar, D. & Castaigne, P. (1980): 'Crossed cerebellar diaschisis' in human supratentorial brain infarction. *Trans. Am. Neurol. Assoc.* **105**, 459–461.

Botez, M.I., Gravel, J., Attig, E. & Vézina, G.L. (1985): Reversible chronic cerebellar ataxia after phenytoin intoxication: possible role of cerebellum in cognitive thought. *Neurology* **35**, 1152–1157.

Botez, M.I., Léveillé, J., Lambert, R. & Botez, Th. (1991): Single photon emission computed tomography (SPECT) in cerebellar disease: cerebello-cerebral diaschisis. *Eur. Neurol.* **31**, 401–412.

Botez, M.I. (1992): The neuropsychology of the cerebellum: an emerging concept. *Arch. Neurol.* **49**, 1229–1230.

De Negri, M., Rolando, S. & Doria, L. (1987): Le atassie infantili. In: *Neurologia infantile*, ed. F. Guzzetta, pp. 371–396. Padova: Piccin.

Feeney, D.M. & Baron, J.C. (1986): Diaschisis. *Stroke* **17**, 817–830.

Gauthier, G.M., Hofferer, J.-M., Hoyt, W.F. & Stark, L. (1979): Visual-motor adaptation. Quantitative demonstration in patients with posterior fossa involvement. *Arch. Neurol.* **36**, 155–160.

Gilbert, P.C.F. & Thach, W.T. (1977): Purkinje cell activity during motor learning. *Brain Res.* **128**, 309–328.

Grafman, J., Litvan, I., Massaquoi, S., Stewart, M., Siriqu, A. & Hallett, M. (1992): Cognitive planning deficit in patients with cerebellar atrophy. *Neurology* **42**, 1493–1496.

Guzzetta, F., Mercuri, E., Bonanno, S., Longo, M. & Spanò, M. (1993): Autosomal recessive congenital cerebellar atrophy. A clinical and neuropsychological study. *Brain Dev.* **15**, 439–445.

Hagberg, B., Sanner, G. & Steen, M. (1972): The dysequilibrium syndrome in cerebral palsy. *Acta Paediatr. Scand.* **61 (Suppl. 226)**, 226–241.

Hart, P.R., Henry, G.K., Kwentus, J.A. & Leshner, R.T. (1986): Information processing speed of children with Friedreich ataxia. *Dev. Med. Child Neurol.* **28**, 310–313.

Holmes, G. (1939): The cerebellum in man. *Brain* **62**, 1–30.

Ito, M. (1990): A new physiological concept on cerebellum. *Rev. Neurol.* **146**, 564–569.

Jervis, G.A. (1950): Early familial cerebellar degeneration (Report of three cases in one family). *J. Ment. Nerv. Dis.* **111**, 398–407.

Kim, S.-G., Ugurbil, K. & Strick, L. (1994). Activation of a cerebellar output nucleus during cognitive processing. *Science* **265**, 949–951.

Lavonde, D.G., Knowlton, B.J., Steinmetz, J.E. & Thompson, R.F. (1987): Classical conditioning of the rabbit eyelid response with mossy-fiber stimulation CS. II. Lateral reticular nucleus stimulation. *Behav. Neurosci.* **101**, 676–682.

Marr, D. (1969): A theory of cerebellar cortex. *J. Physiol.* **202**, 437–470.

Meneghetti, G., Vorstrup, S., Mickey, B., Lindewald, H. & Lassen, N.A. (1984): Crossed cerebellar diaschisis in ischemic stroke: a study of regional cerebral blood flow by 133 Xe inhalation and single photon emission computerized tomography. *J. Cer. Blood Flow Metab.* **4**, 235–240.

Middleton, F.A. & Strick, P.L. (1994): Anatomical evidence for cerebellar and basal ganglia involvement in higher cognitive function. *Science* **266**, 458–461.

Norman, R.M. (1940): Primary degeneration of the granular layer of the cerebellum. An unusual form of familial cerebellar atrophy occurring in early life. *Brain* **63**, 365–370.

Pantano, P., Baron, J.C., Samson, Y., Bousser, M.G., Derouesne, C. & Comar, D. (1986): Crossed cerebellar diaschisis. Further studies. *Brain* **109**, 677–694.

Petersen, S.E., Fox, P.T., Posner, M.I., Mintun, M. & Raichle, M.E. (1989): Positron emission tomographic studies of the processing of single words. *J. Cogn. Neurosci.* **1**, 153–170.

Ryding, E., Decety, J., Sioholm, H., Stenberg, G. & Ingvar, D.F.H. (1993): Motor imagery activates the cerebellum regionally. A SPECT rCBF study with 99mTc-HMPAO. *Cogn. Brain Res.* **1**, 94–99.

Sanes, J.N., Dimitrov, B. & Hallett, M. (1990): Motor learning in patients with cerebellar dysfunction. *Brain* **113**, 103–120.

Weiner, M.G., Hallett, M. & Funkenstein, H.H. (1983): Adaptation to lateral displacement of vision in patients with lesions of the central nervous system. *Neurology* **33**, 766–772.

Chapter 14

The cerebellum contributes to higher cognitive and social behaviour in childhood: evidence from acquired cerebellar lesions

Daria Riva

Divisione di Neurologia dello Sviluppo, Istituto Nazionale Neurologico Carlo Besta, Via Celoria 11, 20133 Milan, Italy

Summary

Many studies have confirmed the role of the cerebellum in the organization of superior brain functions in adults. Congenital cerebellar alterations are frequently observed in children with neurological diseases. These anatomical alterations are associated with neuropsychological or developmental disorders that often give rise to pictures of mental insufficiency of varying severity with behavioral changes even leading to autism. Only few children with acquired cerebellar lesions have so far been described. Here we report 25 children with different kinds of acquired cerebellar lesions (12 with hemispheric astrocytoma, 12 with vermis medulloblastoma, and 1 with hemispheric stroke) who showed different clinical patterns according to the lesion localization. Lesion in the vermis, mainly in the lower lobuli, caused different degrees of behavioral disturbances ranging from irritability to psychosis; lesions in the right hemisphere impaired language processing and symbolic sequencing, categorial memory and executive functions; lesions in the left hemisphere impaired speech prosody, visual sequential memory and design fluency. These data confirm that the connections from the cerebellum to the associative cortical areas are operative very early and that the cerebellum has an essential role in cognitive and social organization also during development.

Very elegant studies of ablative interventions of cerebellum in animals (Down & Moruzzi, 1958) and careful clinical case observations (Holmes, 1930; Amici *et al.*, 1976) followed by more controlled studies on patient populations with cerebellar lesions (Hart *et al.*, 1985; Akshoomoff *et al.*, 1992; Guzzetta *et al.*, 1990), have clearly shown that the cerebellum is essential for the control, integration and learning of motor activities.

This motor control can be highly sophisticated and precise, and the speed of movements very rapid. The motor tasks of the cerebellum can therefore be divided into two activities: on the one hand, it ensures the precise temporal interplay of different set of muscles by means of cerebellar circuits; on the other, it ensures that the movement can be carried out at exceptional speed. This is possible because the cortical structures of the cerebellum are organized in a modular manner which realizes a very regular and crystalline cortical organization. Anatomical evidence for this derives from the fact that cortical cells are organized into longitudinal micromodules, arrayed perpendicularly to the cortical surface and parallel to each other.

It has been shown that the number of these micromodules increased when the cerebellum enlarged, which enlarged the computing capability of the network, which can achieve very powerful computing capability and extraordinary high speed processing and learning (Ito, 1984).

On the other hand, this regular organization suggests that all areas perform a set of similar functions, but that each area performs different functions on a different set of inputs.

Considering that the cerebellum is not necessary for basic perception or for movement, the real role of the cerebellum is to adjust the outputs, both external and internal, to central information, which translates the fact that the cerebellum is a truly associative area.

The projections from the prefrontal, temporo-parietal and paralimbic cortical associative areas through the thalamus are the anatomical substrate that could permit the cerebellum to access information of higher order.

Many PET studies have demonstrated crossed cerebellar diaschisis of two kinds:

- cerebro-cerebellar with metabolic depression in the cerebellar hemisphere contralateral to cerebral supratentorial stroke;
- cerebellar-cerebral with metabolic depression of cortical cerebral areas contralateral to hemispheric cerebellar lesion. Thus the right cerebellar hemisphere is connected with the left cerebral hemisphere and the left cerebellar hemisphere to the right cerebral (Pantano et al., 1986).

The mechanisms used by the cerebellum are very complex and not yet fully understood, but it is also possible that the same mechanisms which regulate complex movements (speed, capacity, consistency) could also regulate cognitive and complex human processes (Schmanhmann, 1991).

To confirm this, there are now a large number of clinical observations of groups and individual patients, and several more sophisticated neuropsychological studies. Clinical studies mainly involving patients with degenerative cerebellar diseases have unexpectedly revealed that they present a vast range of neuropsychological deficits, and that these deficits can be differentiated depending upon whether the ability being tested is processed by the frontal (Luria, 1966; Stuss & Benson, 1986), parietal or occipital areas, or the associative areas (Beyerman, 1917) with which the cerebellum has the greatest number of connections (Ghez & Fahn, 1985).

Patients with agenesia or ipoplasia of cerebellum (Otto, 1873; Doursout, 1891; Bond, 1895), and patients with primarly cerebellar disorders have been studied and the deficits described are rather widely ranging. Patients with Friedreich ataxia have visuo-spatial difficulties, low intelligence IQs and emotional problems (Hart et al., 1985): Olivo-Ponto-Cerebellar Atrophy (Kluin et al., 1988; Kish et al., 1988) patients show different degrees of deficit in verbal and non-verbal intelligence, frontal functions and memory (Bond, 1895). Ataxia-teleangectasia patients show low intelligence (Bond, 1895).

Also in psychiatric patients morphology of the cerebellum is altered: the vermis shows pathological features in a vast majority of schizophrenic patients (Heath *et al.*, 1979). Also in early infantile autism there is a loss of Purkinje cells in lateral and inferior cerebellar cortex and abnormal or reduced number of neurons of fastigial, globose and emboliform nuclei (Ritvo *et al.*, 1986).

More recently precise patterns of neuropsychological malfunctioning were described in patients with focal discrete lesions: this impairment includes mental imagery, anticipatory planning, inability to use temporal cues correctly, visuo-spatial functions and language production.

Lesion of vermis and paravermal structures produce behavioural disturbances, panic and anxiety states, aggressive attitudes (Williams *et al.*, 1980; Courchesne *et al.*, 1988).

The cerebellum is now recognized as playing a much broader role than was thought in the recent past: in connection with the main associative cortical areas, via the thalamus, it is also the refined modulator of complex mental activities, both neuropsychological and emotional.

The aim of this study is to assess different groups of children with different kind of cerebellar lesions in order to verify whether:

(1) also in childhood the cerebellum contributes to higher mental functions;

(2) different localizations of the lesions produce different patterns of impairment;

(3) the connections to cerebral associative areas, particularly the frontal ones, are already established in early age.

To demonstrate the above three points, the following children were evaluated:

– 12 children who underwent surgical resection for cerebellar hemispheric astro- cytoma: five in the left and seven in the right hemisphere;

– eight children who presented, after surgery for medulloblastoma, behavioural disorders of different severity ranging from irritability to a dramatic psychosis;

– one girl with vascular stroke in the right cerebellar hemisphere;

– five children operated upon for medulloblastoma who presented mutism after surgery.

Method

All subjects were studied by neurological examination and MRI.

Neuropsychological assessment included:

(1) observation of spontaneous behaviour

(2) recording of spontaneous language

(3) intelligence evaluation

(4) language evaluation of:

basic receptive and productive abilities

syntactic complex and narrative sentences

computation of mean length utterance (MLU)

(5) memory evaluation

(6) assessment of frontal lobe functions:

    categorial memory

    sequential memory (verbal and visual)

    language fluency

    design fluency (when possible)

    flexibility of reasoning and problem solving

Results and discussion

Astrocytomas (12 children)

Five children underwent surgery for astrocytoma in the left cerebellar hemisphere and seven in the right. Lesions were confined to only one hemisphere, without involvement of the vermis or the contralateral hemisphere. Surgical resection has been completed in all cases. Evaluations were performed twice: one month after the intervention and at least 2 years later.

Results can be summarized as follows:

Children with left hand lesion show impairment of non-verbal intelligence as can be seen in patients with right cerebral hemisphere lesions. They also show a slight aprosody of language and impaired performances in visual sequential memory. Older children perform poorly in design fluency. Lexical (comprehension and production) and syntactic aspects are within normal range.

These results confirm the existence of crossed connections of the left cerebellar hemisphere with the opposite cerebral hemisphere (Pantano et al., 1986) and with the respective supratentorial associative areas (Luria, 1966; Beyerman, 1917). Impairment of non-verbal intelligence is observed in children with right cerebral lesions. The impairment of right cerebral processes is confirmed by the loss of speech melody, which is also processed by right hemisphere.

Lexical competence, also processed in the right hemisphere, is not affected because the healthy opposite left hemisphere compensates. Complex tasks like visual sequential memory and design fluency are processed by frontal lobes – particularly the right. The fact that the activities of the cerebellum are carried out in cooperation with the supratentorial associative areas, in this case with the frontal lobe (right), is confirmed by the defective performance in these specific tasks (Pantano et al., 1986; Luria, 1966; Beyerman, 1917).

Children with right hemispheric lesion show decreased verbal intelligence. Language is very poor with good lexical components (in production and in comprehension). Syntax is on the contrary very defective: the sentences are telegraphic, with very simple association (noun + verb). A severe impairment in sequential verbal and categorial memory is also evident.

Both right and left children show at different degrees impoverished capacities of thinking flexibility and problem solving.

The pictures described are very evident immediately after the intervention. The severity is correlated with the extension of the lesion. Nevertheless the tendency to improvement is very significant, and at mean 2 years after the intervention, even if the specificity of the picture of right or left cerebellar lesion is still recognizable, deficits are very modest and detectable only in laboratory conditions.

Mutism (eight children)

Speech disorders after surgical removal of posterior fossa lesions occur quite frequently. Mutism is less frequent, but is still a not rare event (Ammirati *et al.*, 1989).

The results summarized here derive from the observation of eight children operated upon for medulloblastoma.

In general mutism is considered a 'speech disorder', as a result of dysarthria and to a severe degree of anarthria.

On the contrary we were able to distinguish two main pictures: the first one is the *classical speech disorder* (observed in five children), which consists of a complete anarthria. This disorder refers to a very distinct childhood disorder in which the complete loss of speech evolves to a form of dysarthria. This is described as a syndrome with the following clinical features: (a) occurrence between 2 and 10 years; and (b) transient mutism of variable duration, followed by dysarthria that recovers completely. This condition suggests an extracerebellar component of mutism. Van Dongen *et al.* (1994) describe very well this syndrome, called 'Mutism and Subsequent Dysarthria' (MSD). In his study van Dongen advocates a multifactorial origin of the speech disorder, because the characteristics of speech are not merely pure cerebellar. The most specific features of ataxic speech according to Darley (1969) are 'excess and equal stress' and 'irregular articulatory breakdown' usually not found in these patients.

A possibly more intense manipulation of the brain stem, which can cause ischaemia and possibly oedema, and the involvement of the dentato-thalamic bundles or their cells of origin after surgical intervention in the posterior fossa, are the probable causes.

In general mutism has variable duration, but evolves into a dysarthria that recovers quickly and completely.

The second form is a *real language disorder*. Among the three cases, after the mute phase, we observed language which is usually not dysarthric, but slow and monotonous. This language evolves to a telegraphic and ungrammatical form, with intact comprehension. The characteristics of language are very similar to the language disorders which follow frontal lesions. This kind of deficit improves, but more slowly, and it is accompanied by a vast array of frontal deficits such as impairment of mental flexibility, problem solving, and specifically sequential and categorial memory. This language deficit is associated to lesions localized in the right cerebellar hemisphere, particularly in the lateral neocortex.

Compared with language characteristics of the children operated upon for astrocytoma, the severity is very different: children with medulloblastoma show more dramatic post-operative features, no recovery and a tendency to worsening.

The picture ends in a very hypospontaneous speech. These children prefer not to speak and their poverty of the language is evident also in normal every day life. This can also be due to the invasive nature of the tumour which can destroy the architecture of the cerebellum: some time after the intervention also radiation therapy (with or without chemotherapy) could worsen the deficits, altering the myelin of the axons and thus the connections with the cortical associative areas (Hertzberg et al., 1997).

A 5 years 2 months girl with vascular stroke in the right cerebellar hemisphere

The patient is a right handed girl whose psychomotoric and linguistic development had been completely normal before the onset of the disease. Without any concomitant disease, the girl presented a right cerebellar hemisyndrome with hypothonia, deficient cerebellar coordination and ocular dysmetria. An MRI evaluation revealed a cerebellar stroke involving the posterior part of the right cerebellar hemisphere and partially the cerebellar right basal nuclei. Examinations for screening vascular diseases were negative.

After the acute phase she appeared completely mute and remained in this condition for many days. Two weeks later her ability to understand contextual verbal language was apparently very good and she started to produce isolated words with obvious effort.

After 1 month, her language remained very poor, telegraphic, and reduced to the association between a noun and an uninflected verb, often without functional words.

Anyway the meaning of the linguistic production, even if very poor, was always contextual.

While her intelligence was within normal range, and her comprehension and naming abilities were intact, she was completely unable to put symbols, actions and motor tasks in sequence. Also her verbal sequential memory was very defective. This was evident in spontaneous activities like playing and in laboratory examination. The picture of this child was remindful of that of a 4 years 2 months girl with a viral cerebellitis of unknown origin whom we observed as a first case in which participation of the cerebellum in processing language was suspected (Riva, 1998).

Since the ability of planning and sequential learning is mediated by cerebellar-cortical circuits, particularly those which connect the neocortical structures of cerebellar hemispheres and their associative nuclei (dentate + emboliform) to frontal associative areas 44 + 45 and area 8 via the thalamus (Asanuma et al., 1983; Stanton et al., 1988), also the frontal functions were examined.

On these tests the girl failed, or did very poorly, confirming the malfunctioning of the frontal lobes, particularly of the left.

This picture, even if improved, persists 3 years after onset of the disease and it is mainly characterized by a great slowness in all activities and poor spontaneous language, which even if formally correct was not as rich and fluent as it was before the disease: the patient needs continuously to be encouraged.

Children with behavioural disturbances of different severity (five cases)

These five children affected by medulloblastoma underwent removal of the inferior part of the cerebellar vermis; two of them also underwent surgical ablation of part of the right cerebellar hemisphere.

All of them presented behavioural disorders of different severity: immediately after the intervention, in four, the picture was characterized by strong irritability, reduced (but not abolished) capacity to stay with even familiar persons, and a general attitude to avoid physical and eye contact.

Language was very poorly communicative too, with a tendency to confabulation and iteration. Language components were not impaired to the point of making the meaning of the communication unintelligible, but remained within context and understandable. If anything, language became rather eccentric and bizarre.

In particular, one 9-year-old girl presented after surgery a slight right cerebellar hemisyndrome, but very peculiar behavioural changes: complete gaze aversion, severe intolerance of physical proximity to others, complex rhythmic rocking stereotypes of the trunk and a large amount of linguistic eccentricities.

Her spontaneous language was reduced to extremely rare telegraphic phrases whose content had no relation to the context – often expressed echolalically. Even when encouraged, she tended to repeat individual words out of context in a song-like manner. Her behaviour was frankly psychotic, with elements of disinhibition: she produced swear words and obscenities that were completely unusual before the operation.

No neuropsychological evaluation was possible in the immediate post-operative period because of her behavioural disturbances. After a week the few tests which could be administered revealed a normal lexical and syntactic comprehension, and an extremely severe reduction in categorial fluency: the few words produced were obsessively repeated (foods: 'pasta with ragout', 'pasta with pesto', 'pasta green pasta'); lexical naming prompted invented mechanism. She was not able to put and maintain in sequence motor tasks and other symbolic activities. Her performance on frontal tests was defective. In particular it was impossible for her to find the right strategy to solve several problems. Her graphic abilities had totally disintegrated and she could not even write her own name.

A second evaluation one month later showed clear signs of improvement in all the tests, but she was still deficient for her age. Her behaviour was more composed and more in context, language more structured but still poor: almost all of the stereotypes and prosodic alterations had disappeared.

Two years later her behaviour returned apparently to normal, her language was reasonably fluent without any eccentricities. Nevertheless a frozen attitude and a lack of reciprocity in the social interaction were the main personality characteristics. Her behaviour showed an absence of empathy and a tendency to be on her own.

It needs to be added that the girl in those two years experienced a series of difficult events related to her disease, due to frequent admissions for chemo-radiotherapy; a depressed attitude could be attributed to these circumstances too.

It is difficult to explain why children undergoing a similar operation for the same pathology displayed such a varied range of behaviours. At surgery all cases underwent a more or less complete removal of inferior lobules of vermis. It is possible that subjects undergoing an incomplete removal of inferior vermis display various degrees of irritability, but never full psychosis. This hypothesis is supported by the surgical report and MRI studies that show an incomplete removal of the vermis at operation – on the contrary, a complete removal of the vermis (cerebellar limbic system) from the supratentorial limbic system, leading to psychotic changes of behaviour.

Age can be an important co-factor too. Lastly, fragile psychic organization, relatively compensated within a normal life, based on processing of emotions with instable biological circuits (youngsters are more emotional and passionate) can lead to critical impairment after a devastating experience like surgery of the posterior fossa (Williams *et al.*, 1980; Courchesne *et al.*, 1988).

In such a situation, disruption of functionally active structures for the processing of emotion and relationship adds to the agony which is experienced by the child and the family. Hypoplasia of cerebellar vermis has been documented in psychotic children, confirming the existence of a genetically programmed behavioural regulation. Relational isolation of different entity is found in children with pre-natal abnormalities like vermian hypoplasia (Courchesne *et al.*, 1988; Reiss *et al.*, 1991).

Several progressive systemic diseases in which neurological deficits coexist with mental impairment and social and relational disturbances have shown involvement of the cerebellum, particularly of the vermis (Courchesne *et al.*, 1988; Reiss *et al.*, 1991; Kluin *et al.*, 1988; Kish *et al.*, 1988; Williams *et al.*, 1980; Courchesne *et al.*, 1988).

To conclude, these results seem to confirm the role played in childhood by the cerebellar vermis in controlling social and emotional behaviours.

Conclusions

These results confirm that also at developmental age the cerebellum has an essential role in the organization of higher cerebral functions.

This role is already established from 3 years of age, as demonstrated by our findings, and maybe even earlier considering that congenital partial or total agenesis correlates with poor neuropsychological functioning in many reports.

The internal topographical organization is also confirmed:

- lesions in the vermis, mainly in the lower lobuli, produce different degrees of behavioural disturbances which range from severe irritability to a real picture of psychosis;
- lesions in the right hemisphere produce mainly impairment of language processing and symbolic sequencing, deficits of categorial memory and problem solving;
- lesions in the left hemisphere cause loss of speech melody, impaired fluency of designs and deficits in visual sequential memory.

These data prove that:

- the connections from the cerebellum to the associative cortical areas (particularly the frontal ones) and vice-versa, are established very early in life; and
- the persistence of these deficits over time demonstrates that plastic reorganization of the young brain is not so powerful as to fully compensate even very early lesions (Riva, 1998).

References

Akshoomoff, N.A., Courchesne, E., Press, G.A. & Iragui, V. (1992): Contribution of the cerebellum to neuropsychological functioning: evidence from a case of cerebellar degenerative disorder. *Neuropsychologia* **30**, 315–328.

Amici, R., Avanzini, G. & Pacini, L. (1976): *Cerebellar tumors: clinical analysis and physiopathological correlations*. New York: Karger.

Ammirati, M., Mirzai, S. & Samii, M. (1989): Transient mutism following removal of a cerebellar tumor. *Child Nerv. Syst.* **5**, 12–14.

Asanuma, C. (1983): Distribution of cerebellar terminations to ventral lateral thalamic regions in the monkey. *Brain Res. Rev.* **5**, 237–265.

Beyerman W. (1917): Über angeborene Kleinhirnstörungen. *Arch. Psychiatr. Nervenkr.* **57,** 610–658.

Bond, C.H. (1895): Atrophy and sclerosis of the cerebellum. *J. Ment. Sci.* **41,** 4094–4120.

Courchesne, E., Yueng-Courchesne, R., Press, G.A., Hesselink, J.R. & Jernigan, T.L. (1988): Hypoplasia of cerebellar vermal lobules VI and VII in autism. *N. Engl. J. Med.* **318,** 1349–1354.

Darley, F.L., Aronson, A.E. & Brown, J. (1969): Cluster of deviant speech dimensions in the dysarthrias. *J. Speech Hear. Res.* **12 (3),** 462–496.

Doursout, A. (1891): Note sur quelques cas d'atrophie et d'hypertrophie du cervelet. *Ann. Med. Psychol.* **13,** 345–362.

Down, R.S. & Moruzzi, G. (1958): *The physiology and pathology of the cerebellum.* Minneapolis, MN: University of Minnesota Press.

Ghez C. & Fahn S. (1985): The cerebellum. In: *Principles of neural science,* eds. E.R. Kandel & J.H. Schwartz, pp. 503–522. New York: Elsevier Science Publishers.

Guzzetta F., Mercuri, E., Bonanno, S., Longo, M. & Spanò, M. (1990): Autosomal recessive congenital atrophy. A clinical and neuropsychological study. *Brain Dev.* **15,** 439–445.

Hart, R.O., Kwentus, J.A., Leshner, R.T. & Frazier, R. (1985): Information processing speed in Friedreich's ataxia. *Ann. Neurol.* **17,** 612–614.

Heath, R.G., Franklin, D.E. & Shraberg, D. (1979): Gross pathology of the cerebellum in patients diagnosed and treated as functional psychiatric disorders. *J. Nerv. Ment. Dis.* **167,** 585–592.

Hertzberg, H., Huk, W.J., Ueberall, M.A., Langer, T., Meirer, W., Dopfer, R., Skalej, M., Lackner, H., Bode, U., JanBen, G., Zintl, F. & Beck, J.D. (1997): CNS late effects after ALL therapy in childhood. Part I: Neuroradiological findings in long-term survivors of childhood ALL – an evaluation of the interferences between morphology and neuropsychological performance. *Med. Pediatr. Oncol.* **28,** 387–400.

Holmes, G. (1930): The cerebellum of man. *Brain* **62,** 1–30.

Ito, M. (1984): *The cerebellum and neural control.* New York: Raven Press.

Kish, S.J., El-Awar, M., Schut, L., Leach, L., Oscar-Beramn, M. & Freedman, M. (1988): Cognitive deficits in olivopontocerebellar atrophy: implications for the cholinergic hypotesis of Alzheimer's dementia. *Ann. Neurol.* **24,** 200–206.

Kluin, K.J., Gilman, S., Markel, D.S., Koeppe, R.A., Rosenthal, G. & Jumck, L. (1988): Speech disorders in olivopontocerebellar atrophy correlate with positron emission tomography findings. *Ann. Neurol.* **23,** 547–554.

Luria, A.R. (1966): *Higher cortical functions in man.* New York: Basic Books.

Otto, A. (1873): Ein Fall von Verkümmerung des Kleinhirns. *Arch. Neurosci.* **4,** 730–746.

Pantano, P., Baron, J.C., Samson, Y., Bousser, M.G., Derousne, C. & Comar, D. (1986): Crossed cerebellar diaschisis. *Brain* **109,** 677–694.

Reiss, A.L., Aylward, E., Freund, L.S., Joshi, P.K. & Bryan, R.N. (1991): Neuroanatomy of fragile X syndrome: the posterior fossa. *Ann. Neurol.* **27,** 223–240.

Ritvo, E.R., Freeman, B.J. & Scheibel, A.B. (1986): Lower Purkinje cell counts in the cerebella of four autistic subjects: initial findings of the UCLA-NSAC autopsy research report. *An. J. Psychiatr.* **143,** 8.

Riva, D. (1998): The cerebellar contribution to language and sequential functions: evidence from a child with cerebellitis cortex. *Cortex* **34,** 279–287.

Schmahmann, J.D. (1991): An emerging concept. The cerebellar contribution to higher function. *Arch. Neurol.* **48,** 1178–1187.

Stanton, G.B., Goldberg, M.E. & Bruce, J. (1988): Frontal eye fields efferents in the macaque monkey: subcortical pathways and topography of striatal and thalamic terminal fields. *J. Comp. Neurol.* **271 (4),** 473–492.

Stuss, D.T. & Benson, D.F. (1986): *The frontal lobes.* New York: Raven Press.

Van Dongen, H., Catsman-Berrevoets, C.E. & Van Mourik, M. (1994): The syndrome of cerebellar mutism and subsequent dysarthria. *Neurology* **44,** 2040–2046.

Williams, R.S., Hauser, S.L., Purpura, D.P., Delong, G.R. & Swisher, C.N. (1980): Autism and mental retardation. *Arch. Neurol.* **37,** 749–753.

Index

Page numbers in italics refer to figures or illustrations

A

acallosal children 24, 27, 48–49, 138
  hemispheric specialization 23–30
  interhemispheric communication 35–38
  see also corpus callosum
acquired childhood aphasia 69–76, *75*
adaptation to novel situations 135, 137, 149
agenesis of the corpus callosum *see*
  acallosal children
agnosias 47, 109–118
agraphia 63
akinetopsia 82
alexia 44–45, 49–50, 52
amnesia 16, 47, 114
see also memory
amygdala 17, 19
anarthria 155
anomia 44–45, 49–50, 52, 61–62
anterior commissure 29–30, 38, 48
anterograde amnesia 15–17
aphasia 4–7, 9–10, 68
  lesion localisation 67–76
  subcortical lesions 59–64, *60*
apperceptive agnosia 109–112
apraxia 5, 9, 44–45, 49, 52
archicerebellum 145
associative agnosia 109–110, 112–114
associative areas 151–152, 155, 158
astrocytoma surgery 153–154

asymmetry of hemispheric function *see*
  hemispheric specialization
asynergia 146
ataxi 146, 147, 155
attention 84–88, 99
  and the split-brain 50–52, *51*
auditory comprehension 60, 62, *68*, 69
auditory perception, and BPPD 134
autism 18, 152

B

Balint's syndrome 84, 87–88
basal ganglia lesions 57–64
basic phonological processing
  disorder 133–134, *134*
behaviour 58–59, 63, 99
cerebellum and 152, 156–158
closed head injury and 105–106
bilateral representation 92
duplication in acallosal children 23, 27–30
see also lateralization; symmetrical
  hemispheric function
blindsight 46–47
brain anatomy 57–58
see also hemispheric specialization;
  localization
brain damage
  and language development 121–130
  see also closed head injury
brain plasticity 37, 121–122, 158

Broca's area 10, 62

C
callosal agenesis *see* acallosal children
callosal resection 42–44, *44–45, 48*, 89
caudate nucleus 57, 63
cerebellar infarction 148, 155–156
cerebellum
 acquired lesions and higher
  behaviour 151–158
 congenital lesions 145–149
cerebral cortex *see* hemispheric
 specialization; localization
cerebral insults *see* strokes (insults)
children 5, 9
see also development
 closed head injury 97–107, *102–103,
  105–106*
 cognitive development 58–59
 frontal lobe lesions in 97–107, *104*
 cerebellum in 146–149, 151–158
 commissures 29–30, 38, 41–42, 48, 50
 spatial attention 87–88
 see also corpus callosum
communication *see* interhemispheric
 communication; language
compensation 18, 46, 158
 acallosal children 29, 30, 36–38
 comprehension 60, 62, *68*, 69, 123–124
 concept formation skills 135
 congenital aphasia 69
 congenital lesions of cerebellum 145–149
 congenital prosopagnosia 118
corpus callosum 23, 29–30, 37–38
 acquired lesions 41–52
 see also acallosal children
cortex *see* hemispheric specialization;
 localization
cortical dysplasia 149
crossed aphasia 9, 71
crossed cerebellar diaschisis 147–148,
 152, 154
crossed-uncrossed difference 37–38,
 47–50, *48*

D
declarative memory 15–16

design fluency 154
development
 and white matter model 137–138
 cerebellum and 146–148
 memory and 15–20
 see also children; cognitive development;
  language development
developmental agnosia 116–118
developmental aphasia 69–70
developmental dyslexia 7, 9
developmental prosopagnosia 117
dichaptic tactile procedures 25–26, *25, 27*
disconnection syndrome 36–37,
 42–47, 49–50
discourse *see* narrative discourse
disequilibrium syndrome 146
dorsal visual pathway 80, *80–88*
duplication of functions 23, 27–30
dysarthria 155
dyspraxia 45, *45*

E
early brain damage and language
 development 121–130
embryology of cerebellum 145–146
emotional behaviours 157–158
epilepsy 17, 19, 116
 callosal resection 42–44, *44*
equipotentiality 121
executive functions 98–101, *101–102*, 107
facial recognition 117
 see also information processing
explicit memory 15–16
expressive aphasia *see* nonfluent aphasic
 patients
extinction (hemispatial inattention) 86
extrafrontal regions *102, 104*

F
facial recognition 114–118, *115*
filtering operations 89
fissurae 145
flexibility of the brain *see* plasticity
flexible thinking 154
fluent aphasic patients 60–61, 69,
 71–76, *72– 75*
Friedreich ataxia 147–148, 152

frontal lobes	6–7, 9, 97–98, 123	basic phonological processing	
and cerebellar lesions	153–156	disorder	133–134, *134*
cognitive deficit after injury	97–107, *102, 104–105*	cerebellar lesions	154–157
		closed head injury	106–107
		early brain damage	121–130
G		NLD syndrome	137
gist information	106–107	*see also* aphasia	
global-local processing tasks	88, 88–92, *90–91*	language development	3–4, *4*, 76, 121–124, *123*, 126–130
grammatical morphology	126–127, *126–127*, 130	role of cerebellum	148–149
		strong in NLD	135
		see also speech	
H		lateralization	28
head injury, closed	97–107, *102–103, 105–106*	dorsal visual pathway	81–88
		ventral visual pathway	88–92
hemialexia	36–37	*see also* bilateral representation; hemispheric specialization	
hemianomia	36–37		
hemispatial neglect	86–87	learning disabilities	17
hemispheric separation	46–50	non-verbal	133–140, *136*
hemispheric specialization	5–10, *8*, 18	left hemisphere	4, 5, 9, 28
acallosal children	23–30	cerebellar lesions	154, 158
attention	50–52	language and	68, 122–125, *125*, 134
language development	123–124	subcortical lesions	59–63
see also lateralization; left hemisphere; right hemisphere		visuospatial information processing	79–92
		see also hemispheric specialization	
hierarchical organization of		lesions *see* localization	
spatial processing	88, 88–91	limbic seizures	17, 19
higher cognitive and social behaviour	151–158	linguistic deficits *see* language deficits	
higher-order perceptual processes	89	linguistic development *see* language development	
hippocampus, and memory	16–20		
I		local-global processing tasks	88, 88–92, *90–91*
immature brain plasticity	37, 121–122, 158	localization of function	1–11, *4*
information processing	47, 52	aphasia	67–76, *75*
cerebellum in	147, 149	compensation	18
visuospatial	50, 79–92	language	62, 122, 130
see also executive functions		*see also* hemispheric specialization	
inhibitory control	99–101, *102*	location of objects	83–84
integrative deficits	111–112, 128	long-term memory	16
interhemispheric communication	35–38, 46–47, 49		
		M	
ipsilateral pathways	29, 37–38, 46	medulloblastoma surgery	153–157
irritability	157	memory	15–20, 47
		knowledge of objects	113–114
L		spatial location	83–84
language deficits	18	mental blindness	109–110
basal ganglia lesions	57–64	mental retardation	148–149

see also cognitive development
morphology, grammatical 126–127, *126–127*, 130
motion detection 47, 81–83
motor aphasia *see* nonfluent aphasic patients
motor responses 146–149, 151
corpus callosum and 37–38, 45, 48–50
NLD syndrome 137
subcortical lesions 63
mutism 60, 62, 153–156

N

narrative discourse 124–125, *125–126*, 128–130
after closed head injury *106*, 106–107
neglect 47, 86–87
neocerebellum 145–146
neocortex, and memory 16–17, 20
neuroplasticity *see* plasticity
neuropsychological dysfunction and basal ganglia lesions 57–64
newborn babies, facial recognition 116–117
nonfluent aphasic patients 60–62, 69–76, *72–74*
non-verbal learning disabilities 133–140, *136, 138–139*
non-verbal tasks 4
acallosal children 25, 25–28, 45
cerebellar lesions 154
novel situations, adaptation to 135, 137

O

object-based attention 86–88
object location 83–84
object recognition 111, 113–114, 116–118
global-local processing tasks 90
see also agnosias
object tracking 47, 81–83
occipital lobe 82–84, 111
occipitotemporal regions 90, 113, 116
oculomotor responses 50
organization of memory *see* memory

P

paleocerebellum 145–146
parahippocampal region 16–17, 19–20
parietal lobe 82–86, 88, 110, 112

part-whole distinction in visual perception 88
perceptual processes 109–112, 114, 117
disunity 50
global-local processing tasks 89
role of cerebellum 149
tactile-perceptual performance 133, 135, 137
personal identity node 116, 118
personality *see* behaviour
phonological processing
disorder 133–134, *134*
planning capacity 99–100, *101*
role of cerebellum 147, 149
plasticity of immature brain 37, 121–122, 158
plasticity of language development 130
Poffenberger paradigm 48–49
Posner model of attention 85
posterior brain areas 60–62, 75–76
prefrontal cortex 83–84, 97–100, 103–106
premotor area 84
problem solving 99, 100–101, *101*
cerebellar lesions and 154
non-verbal 135
prosopagnosia 114–118
psychiatric patients 152
psychomotor performance 133, 135, 137
psychotic children 157

R

reading disability 7, 9
receptive aphasia *see* fluent aphasic patients
receptive field hypothesis 86
recognition deficits *see* agnosias
relational disturbances 157–158
representations 99, 112, 115–116
resource allocation 99
right hemisphere 6–9, *8*
acallosal children 23, 28
cerebellar lesions 154, 158
language and 123–125, *125*, 128–130, 158
non-verbal learning disabilities 138, 140
subcortical lesions 63–64
see also hemispheric specialization
rote learning 135–137

S

seizures *see* epilepsy
selection negativity 89

self regulation	100
semantic access agnosia	113–114
semantic information	112–114
facial recognition	116, 118
parahippocampal region and	16
sensory aphasia *see* fluent aphasic patients	
sensory processing, and agnosias	110
sentences *see* syntax	
severity of injury	*103*, 103–106
shape agnosia	111
simultanagnosia	116
social behaviour	
NLD syndrome	136–137
role of cerebellum	151–158
space-based attention	86–88
spatial information processing	79–92
see also non-verbal tasks; visuospatial performance	
specialization *see* hemispheric specialization	
speech	4, 10, *72*, 123–124
fluent/nonfluent division	69, 72, *72*
mutism	60, 62, 153–156
see also aphasia; language	
speech rate	71–74, *74*
splenium	49–50
split-brain patients	36, 37, 45–46, 48–52
spatial information processing	89
split-chiasm animals	42–44
stimulus analysis *see* associative agnosia	
story telling *see* narrative discourse	
strokes (insults)	58–59, 121, 123–124, 148
cerebellar	148, 155–156
subcortical lesions	58–64, *60*, 68–69, 76
superior temporal gyrus	89
superior temporal sulcus	116
supratentorial areas	146, 154
symmetrical hemispheric function	27, 29, 42
see also bilateral representation	
symmetrical theory of hemispheric dominance	5
syntax, complex	127–128, *128*, 130

T

tachistoscopic procedures	26, *27*, 36, 44–45
tactile-perceptual performance	133, 135, 137
tactuomotor learning	37, 46
target detection	85–86
temporal lobe	89–90, 117, 124, *126*, 127
temporal organization of behaviour	99
temporo-mesial structures, and memory	15–20
temporoparietal injury	86
time, sense of	135
transformational agnosia	112

U

uncrossed responses *see* crossed-uncrossed difference

V

vascular stroke *see* strokes (insults)	
ventral visual pathway	*80*, 80–81, 88–92
verbal memory	156
verbal tasks	134, 136–137
acallosal children	25–28
cerebellar lesions and	154
vermis	145, 146, 152, 157–158
visual memory	114, 116, 154
visual perception	45–47, *80*
developmental agnosia	117
global-local processing tasks	88–90, *90–91*
split-brain patients	50
subcortical lesions	63
see also spatial information processing	
visual search	85–86
visuomotor responses	37–38, 49–50
visuospatial performance	6, 8, 133, 135, 137
left hemisphere	79–92
role of cerebellum	147, 149
subcortical lesions	63

W

Wernicke's aphasia	10, 60, 62
white matter model	137–138, *138–139*, 140
whole-part distinction in visual perception	88
word production	123–124
working memory	99–100
writing disorders	63